Letters on t

Containing ample evidence that ......

whatever name known, cannot be transmitted from the

persons of those labouring under it to other individuals

William Fergusson and J. Gillkrest

Alpha Editions

This edition published in 2022

ISBN : 9789356783140

Design and Setting By
Alpha Editions
www.alphaedis.com
Email - info@alphaedis.com

As per information held with us this book is in Public Domain.
This book is a reproduction of an important historical work. Alpha Editions uses the
best technology to reproduce historical work in the same manner it was first
published to preserve its original nature. Any marks or number seen are left
intentionally to preserve its true form.

Contents

LETTERS ON THE CHOLERA MORBUS;

SHEWING THAT IT IS

NOT A COMMUNICABLE DISEASE.

-

LETTER I.

If we view the progress of this terrific malady, as it tends to disorganise society wherever it shows itself, as it causes the destruction of human life on an extensive scale, or as it cramps commerce, and causes vast expense in the maintenance of quarantine and cordon establishments, no subject can surely be, at this moment, of deeper interest. It is to be regretted, indeed, that, in this country, political questions (of great magnitude certainly), should have prevented the legislature, and society at large, from examining, with due severity, all the data connected with cholera, in order to avert, should we unhappily be afflicted with an epidemic visitation of this disease, that state of confusion, bordering on anarchy, which we find has occurred in some of those countries where it has this year appeared.

Were this letter intended for the eyes of medical men only, it would be unnecessary to say that, during epidemics, the safety of thousands rests upon the solution of these simple questions:—Is the disease communicable to a healthy person, from the body of another person labouring under it, either *directly*, by touching him, or *indirectly*, by touching any substance (as clothes, &c.) which might have been in contact with him, or by inhaling the air about his person, either during his illness or after death?—Or is it, on the other hand, a disease with the appearance and progress of which sick persons, individually or collectively, have no influence, the sole cause of its presence depending on unknown states of the atmosphere, or on terrestrial emanations, or on a principle, *aura*, or whatever else it may be called, elicited under certain circumstances, from both the earth and air?—In the one case we have what the French, very generally I believe, term *mediate* and *immediate* contagion, while the term *infection* would seem to be reserved by some of the most distinguished of their physicians for the production of diseases by a deteriorated atmosphere:—much confusion would certainly be avoided by this adoption of terms.[1] Now it is evident, that incalculable mischief must arise when a community acts upon erroneous decisions on the above questions; for, if we proceed in our measures on the principle of the disease not being either directly or indirectly transmissible, and that it should, nevertheless, be so in fact, we shall consign many to the grave, by not advising measures of separation between those in health, and the persons, clothes, &c., of the sick. On the other hand, should governments and the heads of families, act on the principle of the disease being transmissible from person to person, while the fact may be, that the disease is produced in each person by his breathing the deteriorated atmosphere of a certain limited surface, the calamity in this case must be very great; for, as has happened on the Continent lately, cordons may be established to prevent flight, *when flight, in certain cases, would seem to be the only means of safety to many*; and families, under a false impression, may be induced to shut themselves up in localities, where "every breeze is bane."

[1] As medical men in this Country employ the word *infection* and *contagion* in various senses, I shall, generally substitute *transmissible* or *communicable*, to avoid obscurity.

Hence then the importance, to the state and to individuals, of a rigid investigation of these subjects. It is matter of general regret, I believe, among medical men, that hitherto the question of cholera has not always been handled in this country with due impartiality. Even some honest men, from erroneous views as to what they consider "the safe side" of the question, and forgetting that the safe side can only be that on which truth lies (for then the people will know *what* to do in the event of an epidemic), openly favour the side of *communicability*, contrary to their inward conviction; while the good people of the quarantine have been stoutly at work in making out that precautions are as necessary in the cholera as in plague. Meantime our merchants, and indeed the whole nation, are filled with astonishment, on discovering that neighbouring states enforce a quarantine against ships from the British dominions, when those states find that cases of disease are reported to them as occurring among us, resembling more or less those which we have so loudly, and I must add prematurely, declared to be transmissible. It is quite true that, however decidedly the question may be set at rest in this country, our commerce, should we act upon the principle, of the disease not being transmissible, would be subject to vexatious measures, at least for a time, on the part of other states; but let England take the lead in instituting a full inquiry into the whole subject, by a Committee of the House of Commons; and if the question be decided against quarantines and cordons by that body, other countries will quickly follow the example, and explode them as being much worse than useless, as far as their application to cholera may be concerned. It is very remarkable how, in these matters, one country shapes its course by what seems to be the rule in others; and, as far as the point merely affects commerce, without regard to ulterior considerations, it is not very surprising that this should be the case; but it is not till an epidemic shall

have actually made its appearance among us, that the consequences of the temporising, or the precipitation, of medical men can appear in all their horrors. Let no man hesitate to retract an opinion already declared, on a question of the highest importance to society, if he should see good reason for doing so, after a patient and unbiassed reconsideration of all the facts. We are bound, in every way, to act with good faith towards the public, and erroneous
views, in which that public is concerned, ought to be declared as soon as discovered. To show how erroneous some of the data are from which people are likely to have drawn conclusions, is the main cause of my wish to occupy the attention of the public; and in doing this, it is certainly not my wish to give offence to respectable persons, though I may have occasion to notice their errors or omissions.

Previous to proceeding to the consideration of other points, it may be observed, that all doubt is at an end as to the identity of the Indian, Russian, Prussian, and Austrian epidemic cholera; no greater difference being observed in the grades of the disease in any two of those countries, than is to be found at different times, or in different places, in each of them respectively. At the risk of being considered a very incompetent judge, if nothing worse, I shall not hesitate to say, that if the same assemblage, or grouping of symptoms be admitted as constituting the same disease, it may at any time be established, to the entire satisfaction of an unprejudiced tribunal, that cases of cholera, not unfrequently proving fatal, and corresponding in every particular to the average of cases as they have appeared in the above countries, have been frequently remarked as occurring in other countries including England; and yet no cordon or quarantine regulations, on the presumption of the disease spreading by "contagion." For my own part, without referring to events out of Europe, I have been long quite familiar, and I know several others who are equally so, with cholera, in which a perfect similarity to the symptoms of the Indian or Russian cholera has existed: the collapse—the deadly coldness with a clammy skin—the irritability of the stomach, and prodigious discharge from the bowels of an opaque serous fluid (untinged with bile in the slightest degree)—with a corresponding shrinking of flesh and integuments—the pulseless and livid extremities—the ghastly aspect of countenance and sinking of the eyes—the restlessness so great, that the patient has not been able to remain for a moment in any one position—yet, with all this, nobody dreamt of the disease being communicable; no precautions were taken on those occasions "to prevent the spreading of the disease," and no epidemics followed. In the *Glasgow Herald* of the 5th ult., will be found a paper by Mr. Marshall, (a gentleman who seems to reason with great acuteness), which illustrates this part of our subject. This gentleman appears to have had a good deal of experience in Ceylon when the disease raged there, and I shall have occasion to refer hereafter to his statements, which I consider of great value. Nobody can be so absurd as to expect, that in the instances to which I refer, *all* the symptoms which have ever been enumerated, should have occurred in each case; for neither in India nor any-where else could all the grave symptoms be possibly united in any one case; for instance, great retching, and a profuse serous discharge from the bowels, have very commonly occurred where the disease has terminated fatally: yet it is not less certain, that even in the epidemics of the same year, death has often taken place in India more speedily where the stomach and bowels have been but little affected, or not at all. To those who give the subject of cholera all the attention which it merits, the consideration of some of those cases which have, within the last few weeks, appeared in the journals of this country, cannot fail to prove of high interest, and must inspire the public with confidence, inasmuch as they show, *beyond all doubt*, that the disease called cholera, as it has appeared in this country, and however perfectly its symptoms may resemble the epidemic cholera of other countries, *is not* communicable. On some of those cases so properly placed before the public, I shall perhaps be soon able to offer a few remarks: meanwhile, I shall here give the abstract of a case, the details of which have not as yet, I believe, appeared, and which must greatly strengthen people in their opinion, that these cholera cases, however formidable the symptoms, and though they sometimes end rapidly in death, still do not possess the property of communicating the disease to others. I do not mean to state that I have myself seen the case, the details of which I am about to give, but aware of the accuracy of the gentleman who has forwarded them to me, I can say, that although the communication was not made by the medical gentleman in charge of the patient, the utmost reliance may be placed on the fidelity of those details:—

Thursday, August 11th, 1831, Martin M'Neal, aged 42, of the 7th Fusileers, stationed at Hull, was attacked at a little before four A.M., with severe purging and vomiting—when seen by his surgeon at about four o'clock, was labouring under spasms of the abdominal muscles, and of the calves of the legs. What he had vomited was considered as being merely the contents of the stomach, and, as the tongue was not observed to be stained of a yellow colour, it was inferred that no bile had been thrown up. He took seventy drops of laudanum, and diluents were ordered. Half-past six, seen again by the surgeon, who was informed that he had vomited the tea which he had taken; no appearance of bile in what he had thrown up; watery stools, with a small quantity of feculent matter; thirst; the spasms in abdomen and legs continued; countenance not expressive of anxiety; skin temperate; pulse 68 and soft; the forehead covered with moisture. Ordered ten grains of calomel, with two of opium, which were rejected by the stomach, though not immediately.

Eight o'clock A.M. The features sinking, the temperature of the body now below the natural standard, especially the extremities; pulse small; tongue cold and moist; a great deal of retching, and a fluid vomited resembling barley-water, but more viscid; constant inclination to go to stool, but passed nothing; the spasms more violent and continued; a state of collapse the most terrific succeeded. At nine o'clock, only a very feeble action of the heart could be ascertained as going on, even with the aid of the stethoscope; the body cold, and covered with a clammy sweat, the features greatly sunk; the face discoloured; the lips blue; the tongue moist, and very cold; the hands and feet blue, cold, and shrivelled, as if they had been soaked in water, like washerwomen's hands; no pulsation to be detected throughout the whole extent of the upper or lower extremities; the voice changed, and power of utterance diminished. He replied to questions with reluctance, and in monosyllables; the spasms became more violent, the abdomen being, to the feel, as hard as a board, and the legs drawn up; cold as the body was, he could not bear the application of heat, and he threw off the bed-clothes; passed no urine since first seen; the eyes became glassy and fixed; the spasms like those of tetanus or hydrophobia; the restlessness so great, that it required restraint to keep him for ever so short a time in any one position. A vein having been opened in one of his arms, from 16 to 20 ounces of blood were drawn with the greatest difficulty. During the flowing of the blood, there was great writhing of the body, and the spasms were very severe—friction had been arduously employed, and at ten A.M. he took a draught containing two and a half drachms of laudanum, and the vomiting having ceased, he fell asleep. At two P.M. re-action took place, so as to give hopes of recovery. At four P.M. the coldness of the body, discoloration, &c., returned, but without a return of the vomiting or spasms. At about half-past eight he died, after a few convulsive sobs.

On a post-mortem examination, polypi were found in the ventricles of the heart, and the cavæ were filled with dark blood. Some red patches were noticed on the mucuous membrane; but the communication forwarded to me does not specify on what precise part of the stomach or intestinal canal; and my friend does not appear to attach much importance to them, from their common occurrence in a variety of other diseases. It remains to be noticed, that the above man had been at a fair in the neighbourhood on the 9th (two days preceding his attack), where, as is stated, he ate freely of fruit, and got intoxicated. On the 10th he also went to the fair, but was seen to go to bed sober that night. The disease did not spread to others, either by direct or indirect contact with this patient.

Now let us be frank, and instead of temporising with the question, take up in one hand the paper on "cholera spasmodica" just issued, for our guidance, from the College of Physicians by the London Board of Health, and in the other, this case of Martin M'Neal (far from being a singular case this year, in most of the important symptoms),—let the symptoms be compared by those who are desirous that the truth should be ascertained, or by those who are not, and if distinctions can be made out, I must ever after follow the philosophy of the man who doubted his own existence. The case, as it bears on certain questions connected with cholera, *is worth volumes of what has been said on the same subject.* Let it be examined by the most fastidious, and the complete identity cannot be got rid of, even to the *blue* skin, the *shrivelled fingers*, the *cold tongue*, the *change in voice*, and the *suppression of urine*, considered in some of the descriptions to be found in the pamphlet issued by the Board of Health, as so characteristic of the "Indian" cholera; and this, too, under a "constitution of the atmosphere" so remarkably disposed to favour the production of cholera of one kind or other, that Dr. Gooch, were he alive, or any close reasoner like him, must be satisfied, that were this remarkable form of the disease communicable, no circumstance was absent which can at all be considered essential to its propagation. As the symptoms in the case of M'Neal, were, perhaps, more characteristically grouped than in any other case which has been recorded in this country, so it has also in all probability occurred, that more individuals had been in contact with him during his illness and after his death, as the facility in obtaining persons to attend the sick, rub their bodies, &c., must be vastly greater in the army than in ordinary life; so that in such cases it is not a question of one or two escaping, but of *many*, which is always the great test.

Of the College of Physicians we are all bound to speak with every feeling of respect, but had the document transmitted by that learned body to our government, on the 9th of June last, expressed only a "philosophic doubt," instead of making an assertion, the question relative to the contagion or non-contagion of the disease, now making ravages in various parts of Europe, would be less shackled among us. People are naturally little disposed to place themselves, with the knowledge they may have obtained from experience and other sources, in opposition to such a body as the College: but as, in their letter to government of the 18th of June, they profess their readiness, should it be necessary, to "re-consider" their opinion, we, who see reason to differ from them, may be excused for publishing our remarks. It seems surprising enough that, in their letter to government of the 9th of June, the College should have given as a reason for their decision as to the disease being infectious (meaning, evidently, what some call contagious, or transmissible from *persons*)—"having no other means of judging of the nature and symptoms of the cholera than those furnished by the documents submitted to us." Now, according to the printed parliamentary papers, among the documents here referred to as having been sent by the Council to the College, was one from Sir William

Crichton, Physician in Ordinary to the Emperor of Russia, in which a clear account is given of the symptoms as they presented themselves in that country; and, if the College had previously doubted of the identity of the Russian and Indian cholera, a comparison of the symptoms, as they were detailed by Sir William, with those described in various places in the *three volumes* of printed Reports on the cholera of India, in the college library, must at once have established the point in the affirmative. In fact, we know, that the evidence of Dr. Russell, given before the College, when he heard Sir William's description of the disease read, fully proved this identity to the satisfaction of the College. Had the vast mass of information contained in the India Reports, together with the information since accumulated by our Army Medical Department, been consulted, all which are highly creditable to those concerned in drawing them up, and contain incomparably better evidence, that is, evidence more to be relied on, than any which can be procured from Russia or any other part of the world— had these sources of information been consulted, as many think they should in all fairness have been, the College would probably have spoken more doubtingly as to cholera, in any form, possessing the property of propagating itself from person to person. Much of what passes current in favour of the communication of cholera rests, I perceive, on statements the most vague, assertions in a general way, as to the security of those who shut themselves up, &c. To show how little reliance is to be placed on such statements, even when they come from what ought to be good authority, let us take an instance which happened in the case of yellow fever. Doctor, now Sir William Pym, superintendent of the quarantine department, published a book on this disease in 1815, in which he stated, that the people shut up in a dock-yard, during the epidemic of 1814, in Gibraltar, escaped the disease, and Mr. William Fraser, also of the quarantine, and who was on the spot, made a similar statement. Now, we all believed this in England for several years, when a publication appeared from Dr. O'Halloran, of the medical department of Gibraltar garrison, in which he stated that he had made inquiries from the authorities at that place, and that he discovered the whole statement to have been without the smallest foundation, and furnishes the particulars of cases which occurred in the dock-yard, among which were some deaths; this has never since been replied to—so much as a caution in the selection of proofs.

To show, further, how absurdly statements respecting the efficacy of cordons will sometimes be made, it may be mentioned that M. D'Argout, French minister of public works, standing up in his place in the chamber, *on the 3rd instant (Septr.)*, and producing his estimates for additional cordons, &c., stated, by way of proving the efficacy of such establishments, that in Prussia, where, according to him, cordon precautions had been pre-eminently rigorous, and where "*le territoire a été defendu pied à pied,*" such special enforcement of the regulations was attended with "*assez de succès*." in the meantime the next mail brings us the official announcement (*dated Berlin, Sept. 1*) of the disease having made its appearance there!

To conclude, for the present: if there be one reason more than another why the question of cholera should be scrutinized by the highest tribunal—a parliamentary committee—it is, that in the "papers" just issued by the Board of Health, the following passage occurs (page 36):—"But in the event of such removal not being practicable, on account of extreme illness or otherwise, the prevention of all intercourse with the sick, even of the family of the person attacked, must be rigidly observed, unless," &c. There are some who can duly appreciate all the consequences of this; but let us hope that the question is still open to further evidence, in order to ascertain whether it be really necessary that, in the event of a cholera epidemic,

"The living shall fly from
The sick they should cherish."

LETTER II.

In my last letter I adverted to the opinion forwarded to his Majesty's Council on the 9th of June last from the College of Physicians, in which the cholera, now so prevalent in many parts of Europe, was declared to be communicable from person to person. We saw that they admitted in that letter (see page 16 of the Parliamentary Papers on Cholera) the limited nature of the proofs upon which their opinion was formed; but I had not the reasons which I supposed I had for concluding, that because they used the words "ready to reconsider," in their communication of the 18th of same month to the Council, they intended to *reconsider* the whole question. Indeed this seems now obvious enough, as one of the Fellows of the College who signed the Report from that body on the 9th of June (Dr. Macmichael) has published a pamphlet in support of the opinion already given, in the shape of a letter addressed to the President of the College, whose views, Dr. Macmichael tells us, *entirely coincide* with his own; so that there is now too much reason to apprehend that in this quarter the door is closed. Contagionist as I am, in regard to those diseases where there is evidence of contagion, I find nothing in Dr. Macmichael's letter which can make an impression on those who are at all in the habit of investigating such subjects,[2] and who, dismissing such inductions as those which he seems to consider legitimate, rely solely on facts rigorously examined. He must surely be aware that most of the points which he seems to think ought to have such influence in leading the public to believe in the contagion of cholera, might equally apply to the influenza which this year prevailed in Europe, and last year in China, &c.; or to the influenza of 1803, which traversed over continents and oceans, *sometimes in the wind's eye, sometimes not*, as frequently mentioned by the late Professor Gregory of Edinburgh. Who will now stand up and try to maintain that the disease in those epidemics was propagated from person to person? Could more have been made of so bad a cause as contagion in cholera, few perhaps could have succeeded better than Dr. Macmichael, and no discourtesy shall be offered him by me, though he does sometimes loose his temper, and say, among other things not over civil, nor quite *comme il faut*, from a Fellow of the College, that all who do not agree with him as to contagion "will fully abandon all the ordinary maxims of prudence, and remain obstinately blind to the dictates of common sense!"—*fort, mais peu philosophique Monsieur le Docteur.* The time has gone by when ingenious men of the profession, like Dr. Macmichael, might argue common sense out of us; it will not even serve any purpose now that other names are so studiously introduced as *entirely coinciding* with Dr. Macmichael; for, in these days of reform in every thing, *opinions*, will only be set down at their just value by those who pay attention to the subject.

[2] I presume that I shall not be misunderstood when I say, *Would that the cholera were contagious*—for then we might have every reasonable hope of staying the progress of the calamity by those cordon and quarantine regulations which are now not merely useless, but the bane of society, when applied to cholera or other non-contagious diseases.

Referring once more to the Report of the 9th of June, made by the College to the Council, and signed by the President as well as by Dr. Macmichael, the cholera was there pronounced to be a communicable disease, when they had, as they freely admit, "no other means of judging of the nature and symptoms of the cholera than those furnished by the documents submitted to them." The documents submitted were the following, as appears from the collection of papers published by order of Parliament:—Two reports made to our government by Dr. Walker, from Russia; a report from Petersburgh by Dr. Albers, a Prussian physician; and a report, with inclosures, regarding Russian quarantine regulations, from St. Petersburg, by Sir W. Creighton. Dr. Walker, who was sent from St. Petersburg to Moscow, by our ambassador at the former place; states, in his first report, dated in March, that the medical men seemed to differ on the subject of contagion, but adds, "I may so far state, that by far the greater number of medical men are disposed to think it not contagious." He says, that on his arrival at Moscow, the cholera was almost extinct there; that in twelve days he had been able to see only twenty-four cases, and that he had no means of forming an opinion of his own as to contagion. In a second report, dated in April from St. Petersburg, this gentleman repeats his former statement as to the majority of the Moscow medical men not believing the disease to be contagious (or, as the College prefer terming it, infectious), and gives the grounds on which their belief is formed, on which he makes some observations. He seems extremely fair, for while he states that, according to his information, a peculiar state of the atmosphere "was proved by almost every person in the city (Moscow), feeling, during the time, some inconvenience or other, which wanted only the exciting cause of catching cold, or of some irregularity in diet, to bring on cholera;" that "very few of those immediately about the patients were taken ill;" that he "did not learn that the contagionists in Moscow had any strong particular instances to prove the communication of the disease from one individual to another;" and that he had "heard of several instances brought forward in support of the opinion (contagion), but they are not fair ones:" he yet mentions where exceptions seem to have taken place as to hospital attendants not being attacked, but he has neglected to tell us (a very common omission in similar statements), whether or not the hospitals in which attendants were attacked were situated in or near places where the atmosphere seemed *equally productive of the disease in those not employed in attending on sick*. This clearly makes all the difference, for there is no earthly reason why people about the sick should not be attacked, if they breathe the same atmosphere which would seem to have so particular an effect in producing the disease in others; indeed there are good reasons why, during an epidemic, attendants should be attacked in greater proportion; for the constant fatigue, night-work, &c., must greatly predispose them to disease of any kind, while the great additional number always required on those occasions, precludes the supposition of the majority so employed being *seasoned* hospital attendants, having constitutions impenetrable to contagion. Those questions are *now* well understood as to yellow fever, about which so much misconception had once existed. The proofs by disinterested authors (by which I mean those unconnected with quarantine establishments, or who are not governed by the *expediency* of the case) in the West Indies, America, and other places, show this in a clear light; but the proofs which have for some time past appeared in various journals respecting the occurrences at Gibraltar, during the epidemic of 1828, are particularly illustrative. By the testimony of three or four writers, we find that *within certain points*, those in attendance on sick, in houses as well as hospitals, were attacked with the fever, in common with those who were not in attendance on sick; but that, where people remained at ever so short a distance beyond those points, during the epidemic influence, *not a single instance* occurred of their being attacked, though great numbers had been in the closest contact with the sick, and frequently too, it would appear, under circumstances when contagion, had it existed, was not impeded in its usual course by a very free atmosphere:—*sick individuals, for instance, lying in a small house, hut, or tent, surrounded, during a longer or shorter space of time, by their relatives, &c.* A full exposure of some very curious mis-statements on these points, made by our medical chief of the quarantine, will be found from the pen of the surgeon of the 23d regiment, in the *Edinburgh Medical and Surgical Journal*, No. 106.[3] Those who are acquainted with the progress of cholera in India, must be aware how a difference in the height of places, or of a few hundred yards (*indeed sometimes of a few yards*) distance, has been observed to make all the difference between great suffering and complete immunity:—the printed and manuscript reports from India furnish a vast number of instances of this kind; and, incredible as it may appear, they furnish instances where, *notwithstanding the freest intercourse*, there has been an abrupt line of demarcation observed, beyond which the disease did not prevail. A most remarkable instance of this occurred in the King's 14th regiment, in 1819, during a cholera epidemic, when the light company of the regiment escaped almost untouched, owing to no other apparent cause than that they occupied the extremity of a range of barrack in which all the other companies were stationed! so that there would truly seem to be more things "on earth than are dreamt of in the philosophy" of contagionists. This seems so remarkable an event, that the circumstance should be more particularly stated:—"The disease commenced in the eastern wing of the barracks, and proceeded in a westerly direction, but suddenly stopped at the 9th company; the light infantry escaping with one or two slight cases only."—(*Bengal Rep.* 311.) It appears (*loc. cit.*) that 221 attacks took place in the other nine companies. We find (*Bombay Rep.* p. 11.) that, from a little difference in situation, two cavalry regiments in a camp were altogether exempt from the disease, while all the other regiments were attacked. Previous to closing these remarks, which seemed to me called for on Dr. Walker's second Report, it is fair to state, that in certain Russian towns which he names, he found that the medical men and others were convinced that the cholera was brought to them "*somehow or other,*" an impression quite common in like cases, as we learn from Humboldt, and less to be wondered at in Russia than most places which could be mentioned. It will not be a misemployment of time to consider now the next document laid before the College, to enable them to form their opinion,— the Report of Dr. Albers, dated in March, and sent from St. Petersburg;— this gentleman, who was at the head of a commission sent by the Prussian government to Moscow, states, that at St. Petersburgh, *where the disease did not then reign,* the authorities and physicians were contagionists; but at Moscow, where it had committed such ravages, "almost all strenuously maintain that cholera is not contagious." The following extract seems to merit particular attention:—

"When the cholera first reached Moscow, all the physicians of this city were persuaded of its contagious nature, but the experience gained in the course of the epidemic, has produced an entirely opposite conviction. They found that it was impossible for any length of time completely to isolate such a city as Moscow, containing 300,000 inhabitants, and having a circumference of nearly seven miles (versts?), and perceived daily the frequent frustrations of the measures adopted. During the epidemic, it is certain that upwards of 40,000 inhabitants quitted Moscow, of whom a large number never performed quarantine; and notwithstanding this fact, *no case is on record of the cholera having been transferred from Moscow to other places,* and it is equally certain, that in *no situation* appointed for quarantine, *any case of cholera has occurred.* That the distemper is not contagious, has been yet more ascertained by the experience gathered in this city (Moscow). In many houses it happened, that one individual attacked by cholera was attended indiscriminately by all the relatives, and yet did the disease not spread to any of the inmates. It was finally found, that not only the nurses continued free of the distemper, but also that they promiscuously attended the sick chamber, and visited their friends, without in the least communicating the disease. There are even cases fully authenticated, that nurses, to quiet timid females labouring under cholera, have shared their beds during the nights, and that they, notwithstanding, have escaped uninjured in the same manner as physicians in hospitals have, without any bad consequences, made use of warm water used (a moment before) by cholera patients for bathing.

[3] The writer of this, who may be known by application at the printer's, when the present excitement is at an end, is not only prepared to show, *on a fitting occasion*, the correctness of the statements of Dr. Smith as well as those by Dr. O'Halloran just referred to—but also, that in the investigations, in 1828, connected with the question of yellow fever at Gibraltar, facts were perverted in the most scandalous manner, in order to prove the disease imported and contagious:—that individuals had been suborned:—that persons had been in the habit of putting leading questions to witnesses:—that those who gave false evidence have been, in a particular manner, remunerated:—that threats were held out:—and, in short, that occurrences of a nature to excite the indignation of mankind, took place on that occasion; and merited a punishment, not less severe, than a Naval Officer who should give, designedly, a false bearing and distance of rocks.

"These, and numerous other examples which, during the epidemic (we ought, perhaps, to call it endemic) became known to every inhabitant of Moscow, have confirmed the conviction of the non-infectious nature of the disease, a conviction in which their personal safety was so much concerned.

"It is also highly worthy of observation, that all those who stand up for contagion, *have not witnessed* the cholera, which is, therefore, especially objected to their opinion by their opponents." He closes by the observation, "The result of my own daily experience, therefore, perfectly agrees with the above-stated principle, namely, notwithstanding all my inquiries, I *have met with no instance which could render it at all probable that the cholera is disseminated by inanimate objects.*" The words in italics are as in the Parliamentary papers on Cholera, pp. 8 and 9. Here is something to help to guide people in forming opinions, and to help governments on quarantine questions; but owing to a portion of the "perverseness" which Dr. Macmichael in anger talks about, Dr. Albers still *speculates* upon cholera being contagious, and the College, it would seem, take up his speculations and sink his very important facts. Sir William Creighton's Report gives what puports to be an extract from a memorial of his on cholera, given in to the St. Petersburg Medical Council, tending to establish the contagious character of the disease; and with this a report by the extraordinary committee appointed by the Emperor to inquire into the Moscow epidemic. The disease had not appeared at St. Petersburg when he drew up his Memorial, and it does not appear from any-thing which can be seen in the extracts he furnishes, that he had personal knowledge of any part of what he relates. He gives the reported progress of the disease on the Volga and the Don, but is extremely deficient exactly where one might have expected that, from the greater efficiency of police authorities, &c., his information on contagion would have been more precise, viz., the introduction of the disease into Moscow, which could not, it would seem have been by material objects, for, according to the Committee, composed "of the most eminent public officers,"—"the opinion of those who do not admit the possibility of contagion by means of material objects, has for its support both the majority of voices, and the scrupulous observance of facts. The members of the Medical Council have been convinced by their own experience, as also by the reports of the physicians of the hospitals, that, after having been in frequent and even habitual communication with the sick, their own clothes have never communicated the disease to any one, even without employing means of purification. Convalescents have continued to wear clothes which they wore during the disease—even furs—without having them purified, and they have had no relapse. At the opening of bodies of persons who had died of cholera, to the minute inspection of which four or five hours a day for nearly a month were devoted, neither those who attended at their operations, nor any of the assisting physicians, nor any of the attendants, caught the infection, although, with the exception of the first day, scarcely any precautions were used. But what appears still more conclusive, a physician who had received several wounds in separating the flesh, continued his operations, having only touched the injured parts with caustic. A drunken invalid having also wounded himself, had an abscess, which doubtless showed the pernicious action of the dead flesh, but the cholera morbus did not attack him. In fine, foreign *Savans*, such as Moreau de Jonnés and Gravier, who have recognized, in various relations, the contagious nature of the cholera morbus, do not admit its propagation by means of goods and merchandise." (*Parl. Papers on Chol.* p. 13.) With the above documents the Council transmitted to the College a short description of the process of cleaning hemp in the Russian ports; and, lastly, the copy of a letter to the clerk of the Council from our ever-vigilant, though never-sufficiently-to-be-remunerated, head guardian of the quarantine department, who, taking the alarm, very properly recommends, as in duty bound, that a stir be forthwith made in all the pools, and creeks, and bays, &c., of the united kingdom, in order that all those notoriously "susceptible" old offenders, skins, hemp, flax, rags, &c., may be prevented from carrying into execution their felonious intention of covering the landing of a dire enemy. In truth, from the grave as well as from the sublime, there often seems to be "but a step;" and in reading over this gentleman's suggestions about *susceptibles* and *non-susceptibles*, one may fancy himself, instead of being in the land of thinking people, to be in the land of Egypt, where, as we are informed

(Madden, 1825), the sage matrons discuss the point, whether a cat be not a better vehicle for contagion than a dog:—a horse may be trusted, they say, but as to an ass, he is the most incorrigible of contagion smugglers;—of fresh bread we never need be afraid, but the susceptibility of butcher's meat is quite an established thing:—or we might fancy ourselves transported to regions of romance, where it is matter of profound deliberation, whether an egg shall be broken at the large or the small end. Such things are too bad for the nineteenth century; and in England, too, with her enlightened parliament! But until these questions are better examined, our guardian must bestir himself about articles susceptible of cholera contagion, while he enjoys his good quarantine pay, his good half pay from another department as I believe, and withall, if we are not misinformed, a smart pension from the Gibraltar revenue, for what granted nobody can tell.

The documents above referred to, would appear then to be the whole on which the College admit that they formed their opinions, and people may now judge whether the verdict be according to the evidence, or whether it be not something in the *lucus a non lucendo* mode of drawing conclusions:— most persons will probably think that, on such evidence, there might at least have been a qualified opinion. It appears, however, that having come to *a decision* on the 9th of June, that the disease was communicable from person to person, they in three days after, approved of persons being sent to Russia to find out whether they had decided rightly or not. Are we now to expect that, should the occasion need, they will heroically make war against their own declared opinion? For my part I expect from them all that should be expected from men; and the liberal part of the world will not fail to see from this, that I do not despair of even Dr. Macmichael, being still open to conviction. Let it not be for a moment understood that, in any-thing which has been said, or which may remain to be said respecting this gentleman, or in any-thing which may be hereafter said respecting Dr. Bisset Hawkins's work, I mean to insinuate that contagion in cholera is not with them a matter of conscience; but I certainly do mean to say that their zeal has manifestly warped their judgment; and not only this, but that it has prevented them from laying statements before the public on the cholera questions with all the impartiality we might have expected from gentlemen of their character in the profession.

In Dr. Macmichael's pamphlet, consisting of thirty-two pages, and professing to be a consideration of the question, "Is cholera contagious?" we scarcely find the disease mentioned till we come to page 25; the pages up to this being occupied chiefly by a recapitulation of opinions formerly given "on the progress of opinion upon the subject of contagion;"—on the opinions of old writers as to the contagion of plague, small-pox, measles, &c.:—he would infer that whereas small-pox and certain other diseases have, by more accurate observations made in comparatively modern times, been taken from the place they once held, and ranged among diseases decidedly contagious, so ought cholera also to be now pronounced contagious! As an inducement to us to adopt this as good logic, he assures us that the list of diseases deemed contagious by wise men is on the increase—that non-contagionists are *perverse* people, *blunderers*, and so forth! As to his epithets, it shall only be said that among the disbelievers of contagion in cholera, and certain other diseases probably reputed contagious by Dr. Macmichael, are to be found hundreds possessing as much candour, as cultivated minds, and as much practical knowledge of their profession, as any contagionists, whether they be Fellows of a College or not; but as to the statement of Dr. Macmichael, is it true that we have been adding to the list of contagious diseases? Not within the last fifty years certainly. Even the influenza of 1803 was, if I mistake not greatly, termed, very generally, "infectious catarrh," but what professional man would term the influenza of 1831 so? Are there not yet remaining traces of the generally exploded doctrine of even contagion in ague, at one time attempted to be maintained? M. Adouard, of Paris, still indeed holds out. Do we not know that Portal, at one period of his life at least, would not, for fear of "infection," open the body of a person who had died of phthisis? Where is the medical man now to be found who would set up such a plea? or where, except in countries doomed to eternal barbarism, are patients labouring under consumption avoided now, as they were in several parts of the world at one time, just as if they laboured under plague, and all for the simpleton's reason that the disease *often runs through families?* What disinterested man will, on due examination of all that has been written on yellow fever, stand up now in support of its being a contagious disease, of which some thirty or forty years ago there was so general a belief? On croup, and a few more diseases, many still think it *wise to doubt.* Is dysentery, known to make such ravages sometimes, especially in armies, considered now, as at one time, to be contagious? If Dr. Macmichael's pamphlet was intended altogether for readers not of the profession, *which seems very probable*, his purposes will perhaps be answered, at least for a time, but I do not see how it can make an impression on medical men. Why not have been a little more candid when quoting Sydenham on small-pox, &c. and have quoted what that author says of the disease which he (Dr. M.) professes to write about,—the cholera? The public would have means of judging how far the disease which was prevalent in 1669, resembled the "cholera spasmodica," &c., of late years. Many insist upon an identity (Orton among others), and yet Sydenham saw no reason for suspecting a communicable property. It might have been more to the point had Dr. Macmichael, instead of quoting old authorities on small-pox, measles, &c. quoted some authorities to disprove that Orton and others are wrong when they state it as their belief that some of those old epidemics in Europe, about which so much obscurity hangs, were nothing more or less than the cholera spasmodica. Mead's short sketch of the "sweating sickness" does not seem very inapplicable:—"Excessive fainting and inquietude inward burnings, headach, sweating, vomiting, and diarrhœa."[4] In the letter to the President of the College we see no small anxiety to prove that the malignant cholera is of modern origin also in India, for the proofs from Hindoo authorities, as given in the volume of *Madras Reports*, are slighted. These Reports, as well as those of the other presidencies, are exceedingly scarce, but whoever can obtain access to them will find in the translations at pp. 253 and 255 (not at page 3, as quoted by Dr. Macmichael), enough probably to satisfy him that cholera is the disease alluded to there. But I think that we have at page 31 of Dr. Macmichael's letter, no small proof of a peculiarity of opinion, when we find that he there states that the evidence in the *Madras Reports* of the existence of epidemics of malignant cholera in India, on several occasions previous to 1817, rests on imperfect records, and that the description of the disease is too vague to prove the identity with the modern spasmodic cholera; for in this opinion he seems, as far as I have been able to discover, to stand alone among writers on cholera;—indeed it seems established, *on the fullest authority*, that cholera, in the same form in which it has appeared epidemically of late years, has committed ravages in India on more than one occasion formerly:—this is fully admitted by Mr. Orton, an East India practitioner, who is one of the few contagionists.

[4] If the progress of the sweating sickness was similar to that of cholera, the advice of the King to Wolsey was sound; for instead of recommending him to rely on any-thing like cordon systems, or to shut himself up surrounded by his guards, he tells him (see *Ellis's* letters) to "fly to *clene* air incontinently," on the approach of the disease. I use the words *approach of the disease* occasionally, as it is a manner of expression in general use, but it is far from being strictly applicable when I speak of cholera; *the cause* of the disease it is which I admit travels or springs up at points, and not the disease itself in the persons of individuals, or its germs in inanimate substances.

For one piece of tact the author of the letter deserves great credit; for whereas his College collectively, when forming their opinion on the questions proposed to them by the Council, seemed to throw all India records overboard,—he, in his individual capacity, as author of the letter, sends after them all the Russian reports in support of contagion; for anxious as he is to prove his point, not a word do we get of the *on dits* so current in Russia about persons being attacked with the disease from smelling to hemp arrived from such or such a place; from having looked at a boatman who had been up the Volga or down the Volga, &c. &c.: all which statements, when duty inquired into, prove to be unsupported by any thing in the shape of respectable authority, and this is now, in all probability, pretty generally known to be the case, as Dr. Macmichael must be quite aware of.

To the medical gentlemen of India who have been concerned in the official reports, which do them, *en masse*, so much credit, Dr. Macmichael is little disposed to be complimentary; and, indeed, he seems to insinuate that those were rather stupid fellows who did not come to what he is pleased to consider "a just and right conclusion," as to contagion; he thinks, however, that he has got a few of "the most candid" to join in his belief. We shall see whether he had better reason to look towards the Ganges and Beema for a confirmation of his doctrines, than he had toward the Don or the Volga. How does the case stand with respect to one of the gentlemen whom he quotes,—Mr. Jukes, of the Bombay Establishment? This gentleman, like all who speak of cholera, mentions circumstances as to the progress of the disease which he cannot comprehend, and Dr. Macmichael shows us what those circumstances are; but Dr. Macmichael does not exhibit to us *what does* come perfectly within Mr. Jukes's comprehension, but which is not quite so suitable to the doctor's purpose. This omission I shall take the liberty to supply from an official letter from Mr. Jukes in the Bombay Reports:—"I have had no reason to think it has been contagious here, neither myself nor any of my assistants, who have been constantly amongst the sick, nor any of the hospital attendants, have had the disease. It has not gone through families when one has become affected. It is very unlike contagion too, in many particulars." &c.—(*Bombay Reports*, page 172.)— Ought we not to be a little surprised that so great an admirer of candour, as Dr. Macmichael seems to be, should, while so anxious to give every information to his readers, calculated to throw light upon the subject of cholera, omits the above important paragraph, which we find, by the way *immediately precedes* the one upon opinions and difficulties which he quotes from the same gentleman? But let us examine what the amount of force is, which can be obtained from that part of Mr. Jukes's paper, which it does please Dr. Macmichael to quote:—"If it be something general in the atmosphere, why has it not hitherto made its appearance in some two distinct parts of the province at the same time? Nothing of this kind has, I believe, been observed. It still seems creeping from village to village, rages for a few days, and then begins to decline." I find myself unable, at this moment, to ascertain the extent of Mr. Jukes's means of obtaining information as to what was passing in other parts of his province; but I think the following quotation, on which I am just now able to lay my hand, will not only satisfactorily meet what is here stated, but must, in the public opinion, be treasured, as it serves at once to displace most erroneous ideas long prevalent, and which, I believe, greatly influenced men's decisions as to contagion:—"It may, then, first be remarked, that the rise and progress of the disorder were attended by such circumstances as showed it to be entirely independent of contagion for its propagation. Thus we have seen that it arose at nearly one and the same time in many different places, and that in the same month, nay, in the same week, it was raging in the unconnected and far-distant districts of Behar and Dacca." (Bengal Reports, p. 125.) Again (p. 9), that in Bengal "it at once raged simultaneously in various and remote quarters, without displaying a predilection for any one tract or district more than for another; or any thing like regularity of succesion in the chain of its operations." In support of what is stated in these extracts, the fullest details are given as to dates and places; and at page 9 of those Reports, a curious fact is given, "That the large and populous city of Moorshedabad, from extent and local position apparently very favourably circumstanced for the attacks of the epidemic, should have escaped with comparatively little loss, whilst all around was so severely scourged." This seems to have been pretty similar to what is now taking place with respect to the city of Thorn, which remains free from cholera, though the communication is open with divers infected places in every direction. Should Thorn still be attacked by the disease (as it sooner or later will, in all human probability), the contagionists *par métier* will try to establish a case of hemp or hare-skin importation, I have no doubt. I wonder much that Dr. Macmichael or Dr. B. Hawkins, when favouring us with eastern quotations, did not give the public the opinion of Dr. Davy, who is so well known in Europe, and who saw the cholera in Ceylon; his conjecture (quite accessible, I believe, to every medical man in London) may perhaps be as valuable as that of any other person. The following is a copy of it:—"The cause of the disease is not any sensible change in the atmosphere; yet, considering the progress of the disease, its epidemic nature, the immense extent of country it has spread over, we can hardly refuse to acknowledge that its cause, though imperceptible, though yet unknown, does exist in the atmosphere. It may be extricated from the bowels of the earth, as miasmata were formerly supposed to be; it may be generated in the air, it may have the properties of radiant matter, and, like heat and light, it may be capable of passing through space unimpeded by currents; like electricity, it may be capable of moving from place to place in an imperceptible moment of time." Dr. Davy is an army physician, and the report of which this is an extract, may be seen at the Army Medical Office, a place which, of late years, has become a magazine of medical information of the most valuable kind in Europe. There is this difference between army and other information on cholera, that (whether in the King's or E. I. Company's service) the statements given by the medical gentlemen have their accuracy more or less guaranteed by a certain system of military control over the documents they draw up: thus, in the circumstance already noticed as having occurred in the 14th regiment, we have every reason to rely upon its accuracy, which we could not have in a similar statement among the population of any country; and we have, I think, no reason to believe that in pronouncing the cholera of Ceylon not contagious, Dr. Davy, as well as two other gentlemen of high character and experience (Drs. Farrel and Marshall), have not gone upon such data as may bear scrutiny.

LETTER III.

Having given, in my last letter, Dr. Davy's views as to the cause of cholera, I may so far remark just now regarding them, that they are not new, or peculiar to him; and that it may be well, before Dr. Macmichael or others pronounce them vague, that they should inquire whether some of those causes have not been assigned for the production of certain epidemics, by one of the soundest heads of Dr. Macmichael's college—Dr. Prout, who seems, if we have not greatly mistaken him, to have been led to the opinion by some experiments of Herschell, detailed in the Philosophical Transactions of the year 1824. They should recollect that other competent persons devoted to researches on such subjects (Sir R. Phillips among the number) admit *specific local atmospheres* (not at all *malaria* in the usual sense of the term), produced by irregular streams of specific atoms from the interior of the earth, and "arising from the action and re-action of so heterogeneous a mass." For my part I feel no greater difficulty in understanding how our bodies, "fearfully and wonderfully made" as we are, should be influenced by those actions, re-actions, and combinations, to which Sir Richard refers, and of "whose origin and progress the life and observation of man can have no cognizance," than how they are influenced by other invisible agents, the existence of which I am compelled to admit.—If the writer of the article on cholera in the *Westminster Review*, for October, 1831, do not find all his objections met by these observations, I must only refer him to the *quid divinum* of Hippocrates:—but I must protest against logic such has been employed by certain members of our Board of Health, who lately, on the examination of gentlemen of the profession who had served in India, and who had declared the disease not to be communicable, came to the conclusion that it must, nevertheless, be so, as those gentlemen could not show *what it was* owing to.

Most extraordinary certainly it does appear, that while Dr. Macmichael goes to the trouble of giving us (p. 27) the views of *a captain* (!) as to the progress of cholera at a certain place in India, he should have refrained altogether from referring, on the point of contagion or non-contagion, to the report of such a person as Dr. Davy, or to the reports of this gentleman's colleagues at Ceylon, Drs. Farrell and Marshall. Had Dr. Macmichael added a little to his extract from Capt. Sykes, by informing us of what that gentleman states as to the great mortality ("350 in one day") in the town of Punderpoor, "when the disease first commenced its ravages there," people would have means of judging how unlike this was to a contagious disease creeping from person to person in its commencement.

It is painful to be obliged to comment on the manner in which Dr. Bisset Hawkins has handled the questions relative to the Ceylon epidemic, which seems far from being impartial; for, while he quotes (p. 172) Dr. Davy, "a medical officer well known in the scientific world," as stating that the cause of the disease is not in any *sensible* changes in the state of the atmosphere, he breaks off suddenly at the word *atmosphere*, proceeds to talk of the changes in the muscles and blood of persons who die of the disease, and passing over the part quoted from Dr. Davy, near the close of my last letter, Dr. Hawkins leaves his readers to draw a very natural conclusion— that, as Dr. Davy admitted that there were no prevalent *sensible* states of the atmosphere to which the cholera could be attributed, *he, therefore*, believed it to have been propagated by contagion, an inference which we now see must be quite wide of the mark. Dr. Hawkins had, it appears, like many other medical gentlemen, access to the reports from Ceylon, &c., in the office of the chief of the army medical department in London, and it is to be regretted I think that, with respect to one of the Ceylon reports, he only tells us (p. 174) that "Mr. Staff-Surgeon Marshall reports from Candy, that of fifty cases which had occurred, forty died." Why more had not been quoted from a gentleman who had such ample means of witnessing the disease in its very worst form, I must leave to others to say; but, referring again to the highly interesting letter from Mr. Marshall on cholera, which appeared in the *Glasgow Herald*, of the 5th of August last, and in which, from many important observations which every body interested in cholera should read and study, the following remarks will be found:—"In no one instance did it seem to prevail among people residing in the same house or barracks, so as to excite a suspicion that the contact of the sick with the healthy contributed to its propagation." "The Indian Cholera, as it is sometimes called, appears not to be essentially different from cholera as it occurs in this and all other countries." "I consider it, therefore, impossible for a medical practitioner to speak decisively from having seen one, or even a few cases of cholera in this country, and to say whether they are precursors of '*the epidemic* cholera' or not. That the disease is ever propagated by means of personal contact, or by the clothes of the sick, has not, as far as I know, been satisfactorily proved. The quality of contagion was never attributed to the disease in Ceylon, and I believe no-where did it occur in greater severity. I am aware that an attempt has been made to distinguish the ordinary cholera of this country from the 'epidemic cholera,' by means of the colour or quality of the discharges from the bowels. In the former it is said the discharge is chiefly bile, while in the latter it is said to bear no traces of bile, but to be colourless and watery. How far is this alleged diagnosis well founded? I am disposed to believe that, in all severe cases of cholera, whether it be the cholera of this country, or the epidemic cholera, the secretion of bile is either suppressed, or the fluid is retained in the gall-bladder." Mr. Marshall, it may be observed, is the gentleman who was selected by the late Secretary at War, in consequence of his known intelligence, to remodel the regulations relative to military pensioners; and I understand that, in consequence of the manner in which he executed that very important duty, he has since been promoted. After what appears from the above quotations, how perfectly unwarrantable must the assertion of Dr. Bisset Hawkins seem, that "from the Coromandel coast it seems to have been transported by sea to Ceylon!"

We shall, I think, be able to see that the assumption of Drs. Macmichael and Hawkins, as to the importation of the disease into the Mauritius from Ceylon, is equally groundless with that of its alledged importation into the latter island; and here we have to notice the same want of candour on the part of those gentlemen, in not having furnished that public, which they professed to enlighten on the subject of cholera, with those proofs within their reach best calculated to display the truth; be it a part of my duty to supply the omissions of these gentlemen in this respect. The following is a copy of a letter accompanying the medical commission report at that island forwarded to General Darling, the then commanding officer, by the senior medical gentleman there.

"Port Louis, Nov. 23, 1819.

"I have the honour of transmitting the reports of the French and English medical gentlemen on the prevalent disease; both classes of the profession seem to be unanimous in not supposing it contagious, or of foreign introduction. From the disease pervading classes *who have nothing in common but the air they breathe*, it can be believed that the cause may exist in the atmosphere. A similar disease prevailed in this island in 1775, after a long dry season."

(Signed)

W. A. BURKE,
Inspector of Hospitals.

In the reports referred to in the above letter, there is the most ample evidence of the true cholera having appeared at different points in the colony *before the* arrival of the Topaze frigate, the ship *accused* by contagionists *par métier*, of having introduced the disease; so that, contrary to what Dr. Macmichael supposes, those who disbelieve the communicability of cholera, have no necessity whatever in this case for pleading a coinsidency between the breaking out of the disease, and the arrival of the frigate; indeed, his friend Dr. Hawkins seems to be aware of this, when he is obliged to have recourse to such an argument as that "it is, at all events, clear that the disease had not been *epidemic* at the Mauritius before the arrival from Ceylon;" so that the beginning of an epidemic is to be excluded from forming a part or parcel of the epidemic! Why is it that in medicine alone such modes of reasoning are ever ventured upon!

We know, from the history of cholera in India, that not only ships lying in certain harbours have had the disease appear on board, but even vessels sailing down one coast have suffered from it, while sailing up another has freed them from it, without the nonsense of going into harbour to "expurgate." Now, with respect to the *Topaze*, it appears that while lying in harbour in Ceylon, the disease broke out on board her; that after she got into "*clene air*" at sea, the disease disappeared, seventeen cases only having occurred from the time she left the island, and she arrived at the Mauritius, as Dr. Hawkins admits, without any appearance whatever of the cholera on board. On the day after her arrival, she sent several cases ("chronic dysentry, hepatitis, and general debility") to hospital, but not one of cholera; neither did any case occur on board during her stay there, at anchor a mile and a half from shore, and constantly communicating with shore,[5] while a considerable number of deaths took place from cholera *in the merchant vessels anchored near shore.*

[5] Somebody is said to have seen a man on board with vomiting and spasms, on the day before she moved to this anchorage, but the surgeon of the ship has not stated this.

As to the introduction of cholera from the Mauritius into Bourbon, where it appeared but very partially, Dr. Macmichael very properly does not say one word. There was abundance of "precaution" work, it is said, and those who choose, are at liberty to give credit to the story of its having been smuggled on shore by some negro slaves landed from a Mauritius vessel. As to the *precautions* to which the writer in *The Westminster Review* attributes the non-extension of the disease in this island, hundreds of instances are recorded, in addition to those which we have already quoted, of the disease stopping short, without cordons or precautions of any kind—one remarkable instance is mentioned by Dr. Annesley, where, *without seclusion,* the disease did not reach the ground occupied by two cavalry regiments, although it made ravages in all the other regiments in the same camp.

We have, perhaps, a right to demand from those gentlemen who display such peculiar tact in the discovery of ships by which the cholera has, at divers times, been imported into continents and islands, the names of those ships which brought to this country, in the course of the present year, the "*contagion*" which has produced, at so many different points, cases of severe cholera, causing death in some instances, and in which the identity with the "Indian cholera," the "Russian cholera," &c., has been so *perfect*, that all the "perverse ingenuity" of man cannot point out a difference. If it cannot be shown that in this, we non-contagionists in cholera are in error, people will surely see reason for abandoning the cause of cordons, &c., in this disease,—a cause which, in truth, now rests mainly for support upon a sort of conventional understanding, unconnected altogether, it would appear, with the facts of the case, and entered into, we are bound to suppose, before the full extent of the mischief likely to arise from it had been taken into consideration. Admitting for a moment that a case of cholera possessing contagious properties could be imported into this country this year, will anybody say that a "constitution of the atmosphere" favourable to its communicability to healthy individuals, has not existed *in a very high degree*:—can a spot be named in which cholera, generally of a mild grade, has not prevailed? And if contagionists cannot point out a difference between some of the severe cases to which public attention has been drawn, and the most marked cases of the Indian or Russian cholera, I think that now there should be an end to all argument in support of their cause. Without at all going to the extent which might be warranted, I would beg to be informed of the names of the ships by which the contagion was brought, which caused the illness of the following individuals; or if they be allowed, as I presume must be the case, not to have been infected at all in this way, all that has been said regarding the identity of the foreign and severe form of the home disease, must be shown to be without foundation:—the detailed case of Patrick Geary, which occurred in the Westminster Hospital,—the fatal case of Mr. Wright, surgeon, 29, Berwick-street,—the cases, some of them fatal, which occurred at Port Glasgow, and regarding which, a special inquiry was instituted,—a case in Guy's Hospital, which caused some anxiety about the middle of July last,—a case reported in a medical periodical in August last, as having occurred in Ireland,—the fatal case, as reported in my first letter, of Martin M'Neal,[6]— a second case reported in a medical periodical in August,—a fatal case on the 12th of August last at Sunderland, reported upon to the Home Secretary by the mayor of that town,—three cases reported in No. 421 of THE LANCET,—a very remarkable case duly reported upon in September, from the Military Hospital at Stoke, near Davenport, and a case with thorough "congee stools," spasms, &c. (the details of which I may hereafter forward), which occurred at Winchester on the 22d of September, in the 19th Foot, in a man of regular habits, and of *the nature* of which case the medical gentleman in charge had no doubt.

[6] The same Army Medical gentleman, who had been sent to Port Glasgow, was sent to Hull to report upon this case:—he arrived there too late, but having seen the details of the case, he admitted that he saw no reason to declare them different from those which occurred in the Indian cholera.

I quite agree with those who are of opinion, that in this and most other countries, cases may be every year met with exhibiting symptoms similar to those which have presented themselves in any one of the above. Instead of amusing us, when next writing upon cholera, with a quotation about small-pox from Rhazes, bearing nonsense upon the face of it, some of those who maintain the contagious property of Indian or any other cholera, may probably take the trouble to give the information on the above cases, so greatly required for the purpose of enlightening the public.

I must now beg to return to an examination of one or two more of the *very select* quotations made by Dr. Macmichael, with the view, as he is pleased to tell us, of placing the statements on both sides in juxtaposition. He is well pleased to give us from Dr. Taylor, assistant-surgeon,—what indeed never amounted to more than report, and of the truth or falsehood of which this gentleman does not pretend to say he had any knowlege himself,—that a traveller passing from the Deacan to Bombay, found the disease prevailing at Panwell, through which he passed, and so took it on with him to Bombay; but whether the man had the disease, or whether he took its germs with him in some very susceptible article of dress, is not stated by Dr. Taylor; however, he states (what we are only surprised does not happen oftener in those cases, when we consider similarity of constitution—of habits—of site or aspect of their dwellings, &c.) that several members of a family, and neighbours "were attacked within a very short period of each other;" but when Dr. Taylor goes on to say, "In bringing forward these facts, however, it may be proper at the same time to state, that of the forty-four assistants employed under me, only three were seized with the complaint;" he gets out of favour at once, and his observation is called "unlucky," being but a *negative* proof, and Dr. Macmichael adds, what everybody must agree with him in, that positive instances of contagion must outweigh all negative proofs:—to be sure:—but Dr. Macmichael's saying this, does not show that positive proofs exist. Give us but positive proofs, give even but a *few*, which surely may be done, if the disease be really communicable, and where contagion has been so ardently sought after by all sorts of *attachés* and *employés* of the cordon and quarantine systems in the different countries on the Continent. We could produce no mean authority to show, that *a long succession of negative proofs* must be received as amounting to a moral certainty; and what greater proof can we have of non-contagion in any disease, than we have in the fact regarding epidemic cholera, as well as yellow fever, that attendants on the sick are not more liable than others to be attacked? Regard should, of course, always be paid, in taking this point into consideration, to what has been already noticed in my second letter, or the inferences must be most erroneous. Dr. Macmichael quotes the statement of Dr. Burrell, 65th regiment (and takes care to put the quotation in italics too), that at Seroor, in 1818, "almost every attendant in hospital had had the disease. There are about thirty attendants in hospitals." Now, along with hundreds of other instances, what does Dr. French, of the 49th regiment, say, in his Report of 1829? That no medical man, servant, or individual of any kind, in attendance on the sick, was taken ill at Berhampore, when the cholera prevailed there that year, and refers, to his Report for 1825, in which he remarked the same thing in the hospital of the 67th regiment at Poonah; contrary, as he observes, to what occurred some years before in the 65th regiment at Seroor, about forty miles distant. In the two instances quoted by Dr. French, and in that by Dr. Burrell, all those about the sick stood in the same relation towards them, and all the difference will be found probably to have been, that the hospital of the 65th *was within the limit of the deteriorated atmosphere, where the cause existed equally (as in the case of ague and yellow fever) whether persons were present or not.*

In Egypt there is not, it is true, a "cruel and inhuman desertion" of the unfortunate plague patients; for, among other reasons, being predestinarians, they think it makes no sort of difference whether they attend on the sick or not. Those who act upon the principle of cholera being a highly contagious disease, may perhaps consider it necessary to recommend, among their *precautions*, that the medical men and attendants should be enveloped in those hideous dresses used in some countries by those who approach plague patients[7]—fancy, in the case of a sick female, or even of a man of pretty good nerves, the effect of but half the precautions one hears of, as proper to be observed. It is quite a mistake to suppose that the sick have not been sometimes abandoned during the prevalence of epidemics; and that too in cases where medical men had very erroneously voted the disease contagious:—among other horrid things arising out of mistaken views, who that has ever read it, can forget the account given by Dr. Halloran, of the wretched yellow-fever patient in Spain, who, with a rope tied round him, was dragged along for some distance by a guard, when he was put into a shed, where he was suffered to die, without even water to quench his thirst? I admit that, even with the views of non-contagionists, difficulties obviously present themselves in regard to the safety of those about the sick, when the latter are in such a state as will not admit of their removal to a more auspicious spot from that in which there is reason to believe they inhaled the noxious atmosphere. From what has been observed in India and other places, however, there is often sufficient warning in a feeling of *malaise*, &c., and the distance to favoured spots, where people may be observed not to be attacked, may be very short,—sometimes, as we have seen, but a few yards, so that a removal of the patient, *with his friends*, may be practicable, in a vast number of cases, previous to the setting in of the more serious symptoms.

[7] Since writing the above, I find that this scene has actually occurred lately at Dantzic where a few miserable medical men illustrated their doctrines of contagion, by skulking at a certain distance about the sick, dressed up in oil skins, like the disgusting figures we see in books, of the Marseilles doctors in the Lazaretto. (See Sun Newspaper, 22nd, Nov.)

I shall conclude this by cursorily referring to two circumstances which have within a short time occurred on the Continent, and which seem to me to be of no small importance in regard to cholera questions. It appears that the committee appointed by the French Chamber of Deputies to inquire into the questions connected with voting an additional sum to meet cordon and quarantine expenses, in the event of the cholera making its appearance in or near France, have made their report to the Chamber. They declare that in India the cholera was proved not to have been transmissible; and that in regard to Russia, it was not introduced, as always contended for by some persons:—they refer to the city of Thorn as exempt from the disease, though free from cordons, and in the midst of a country where it prevails, while the disease appeared in St. Petersburg and Moscow, notwithstanding their cordons, and even in Prussia, where sanatory laws where executed "*avec une punctualité et une rigeur ailleurs inconnues.*" The money is nevertheless granted; it is always a good thing to have, but they have set one curious *condition* upon its being granted, which displays consummate tact, for it is to be employed solely in disbursements of a particular nature (*dépenses materielles*), including, it may be presumed, temporary hospitals, &c.; and that it is by no means ("*nullement*") to go into the pockets of individuals.

The other circumstance to which I allude is that, like Russia and Austria, Prussia has found that quarantines and cordons do not check the progress of cholera. The king declares that the appearance of the disease in his provinces, has thrown *new light* on the question; he specifies certain restrictions as to intercourse, which were forthwith to be removed, and declares his intention to modify the whole. In short, it is quite plain that, as Dr. Johnson has it in his last journal,—those regulations will, "*in more countries than Russia, be useless to all but those employed in executing them.*"

LETTER IV.

It need scarcely be said how much it behooves all medical men to keep in view the subject of the wide-spreading cholera, and not to suffer themselves to be led from an attentive consideration of all that appertains to it, by the great political questions which at present convulse the whole kingdom.

I totally disagree with Dr. Macmichael, as I believe most people will, that the notion of *contagion* in many diseases is "far from being natural and obvious to the mind;" for, since the time that contagious properties have been generally allowed to belong to certain diseases, there has been a strong disposition to consider this as the most natural and obvious mode of explaining the spreading of other diseases. A person sees evidence of the transmission, *mediate* as well as *immediate*, of small-pox, from one person to another; and, in other diseases, the origin of which may be involved in obscurity, he is greatly prone to assign a similar cause which may seem to reconcile things so satisfactorily to his mind. Indeed there seems, in many parts of the world, a degree of *popularity* as to quarantine regulations, which is well understood and turned to proper account by the initiated in the mysteries of that department:—for what more common than the expression—"we cannot be too careful in our attempts to *keep out* such or such a disease?" For my part, I admit that I can more easily comprehend the propagation of certain epidemics by contagion, than I can by any other means, *when unaccompanied by sensible atmospheric changes*; and if I reject contagion in cholera, it is because whatever we have in the shape of fair evidence, is quite conclusive as to the non-existence of any such principle. Indeed abundance of evidence now lies before the public, from various sources, in proof of the saying of Fontenelle being fully applicable to the question of cholera—"When a thing is accounted for in two ways, the truth is usually on the side most opposed to *appearances*." How well mistaken opinions as to contagion in cholera are illustrated in a pamphlet which has just appeared from Dr. Zoubkoff of Moscow! This gentleman, it appears, has been a firm believer in contagion, until the experience afforded him during the prevalence of the disease in that city proved the contrary. He tells us (p. 10), that in the hospital (Yakimanka) he saw "*to his great astonishment*, that all the attendants, all the soldiers, handled the sick, supported their heads while they vomited, placed them in the bath, and buried the dead; always without precaution, and always without being attacked by cholera." He saw that even the breath of cholera patients was inhaled by others with impunity; he saw, that throughout the district of which he had charge, the disease did not spread through the crowded buildings, or in families where some had been attacked, and that exposure to exciting causes *determined* the attack in many instances. He saw all this, gives the public the benefit of the copious notes which he made of details as to

persons, places, &c., and now ridicules the idea of contagion in cholera. Grant to the advocates of contagion in cholera but all the data they require, and they will afterwards prove every disease which can be mentioned to be contagious. Hundreds of people, we will say, for instance, come daily from a sickly district to a healthy one, and yet no disease for some time appears; but at last an "inexplicable condition of the air," and "not appreciable by any of our senses" (admitted by Dr. Macmichael and others as liable to occur, but *only in aid* of contagion), take place; cases begin to appear about a particular day, and nothing is now more easy than to make out details of arrivals, there being a wide field for selection; and even how individuals had spoken to persons subsequently attacked—had stopped at their doors— had passed their houses, &c.[8] Causation is at once connected with antecedence, at least for a time, by the people at large, who see their government putting on cordons and quarantines, and the most vague public rumour becomes an assumed fact. We even find, as may be seen in the quotation given from Dr. Walker's report, that contagionists are driven to the "somehow or other" mode of the introduction of cholera by individuals; so that it may be deplored, with respect to this disease, in the words of Bacon, that "men of learning are too frequently led, from ignorance or credulity, to avail themselves of mere rumours or whispers of experience as confirmation, and sometimes as the very ground-work, of their philosophy, ascribing to them the same authority as if they rested upon legitimate testimony. Like to a government which should regulate its measures, not by official information of its accredited ambassadors, but by the gossipings of newsmongers in the streets. Such, in truth, is the manner in which the interests of philosophy, as far as experience is concerned, have hitherto been administered. Nothing is to be found which has been duly investigated,—nothing which has been verified by a careful examination of proof."

[8] Since the above was written it has been very clearly shewn how easily proofs of *this kind* may be furnished to all disposed to receive them. We perceive that a disease officially announced as *the true* cholera, has existed for nearly a month past at Sunderland, and that among the thousands of people who left it within that time, nothing could be more easy, had the disease appeared epidemically in other parts of England, than to point out the *particular individual* who had "brought it" in some way or other; and this is the manner in which all the fables about the propagation of cholera from one district to another have gained credence. (Nov. 24th.)

In their efforts to make out their case, there would seem to be no end to the contradictions and inconsistencies into which the advocates of contagion in cholera are led. At one moment we are required to believe that the disease may be transmitted through the medium of an unpurified letter, over seas and continents, to individuals residing in countries widely differing in climate, while, in the next, we are told—regarding the numberless instances of persons of all habits who remain unattacked though in close contact with the diseased—that the constitution of the atmosphere necessary for the germination of the contagion is not present; and

this, although we see the disease attacking all indiscriminately, those who are not near the sick as well as those who are at a very short distance, as on the opposite side of a ravine, of a rivulet, of a barrack, or even of a road. They assume that wherever the disease appears, *three* causes must be in operation—contagion—peculiar states of atmosphere (heat now clearly proved not *essential*, as at one time believed)—and susceptibility in the habit of the individual. However unphilosophical it is held to be to multiply causes, the advocates of contagion are not likely to reduce the number, as this would at once cramp them in their pleadings before a court where sophistry is not always quickly detected. Those who see irresistible motives for dismissing all idea of contagion, look, on the contrary, for the production of cholera, to sources, admitted from remote times to have a powerful influence on our systems, though invisible—though not to be detected by the ingenuity of man, and though proved to exist only by their effects.

Many who do not believe that cholera can be propagated by contagion under ordinary circumstances, have still a strong impression that by crowding patients together, as in hospitals or in a ship, the disease may acquire contagious properties. Now we find that when the *experimentum crucis* of extensive experience is contrasted with the feasibility of this, cholera, like ague, has not been rendered one bit more contagious by crowding patients together than it has been shown to be under other circumstances. We do not require to be told that placing many persons together in ill-ventilated places, whether they labour under ague, or catarrh, or rheumatism, or cholera, as well as where no disease at all exists among them, as in the Calcutta black-hole affair, and other instances, which might be quoted, *fever*, of a malignant form, is likely to be the consequence, but assuredly not ague, or catarrh, or rheumatism, or cholera. On this point we are furnished with details by Dr. Zoubkoff, of Moscow, in addition to the many previously on record. It may be here mentioned that, on a point which I have already referred to, this gentleman says (p. 43), "I shall merely observe that at Moscow, where the police are remarked for their activity, they cannot yet ascertain who was the first individual attacked with cholera.

It was believed at one time that the disease first showed itself on the 17th of September; afterwards the 15th was fixed upon, and at last persons went so far back as August and July." As this gentleman *had been* a contagionist, occupied a very responsible situation during the Moscow epidemic, and quotes time and place in support of his assertions, I consider his memoir more worthy of translation than fifty of your Keraudrens.

Respecting those mysterious visitations which from time to time afflict mankind, it may be stated that we have a remarkable instance in the "*dandy*" or "*dangy*" disease of the West India Islands, which, of late years, has attracted the notice of the profession as being quite a new malady, though nobody, as far as I am aware of, has ever stated it to have been an imported one. We find also that within the last three years a disease, quite novel in its characters, has been very prevalent in the neighbourhood of Paris. It has proved fatal in many instances, and the physicians, unable to assign it a place under the head of previously-described disease, have been obliged to invent the term "Acrodynia" for it. I am not aware that even M. Pariset, the medical chief of quarantine in France, ever supposed this disease to have been *imported*, and to this hour the cause of its appearance remains in as much obscurity among the Savans of Paris, as that of the epidemic cholera.

Considering all the evidence on the subject of cholera in India, in Russia, Prussia, and Austria, one cannot help feeling greatly astonished on perceiving that Dr. Macmichael (p. 31 of his pamphlet) insinuates that the spreading of the disease in Europe has been owing to the views of the subject taken by the medical men of India.

In turning now more particularly to the work, or rather compilation, of Dr. Bisset Hawkins, let us see whether we cannot discover among what he terms "marks of haste" in getting it up for "the curiosity of the public" (*curiosity*, Dr. Hawkins!), some omissions of a very important nature on the subject of a disease respecting which, we presume, he wished to enlighten the public. And first, glancing back to cholera in the Mauritius, Dr. Hawkins might, had he not been so pressed for time, have referred to the appearance of cholera in 1829, at Grandport in that island; when, as duly and officially ascertained, it could not be a question of importation by any ship whatever. The facility with which he supplies us with "facts,"—the *false facts* reprobated by Bacon, and said by Cullen to produce more mischief in our profession than false theories—is quite surprising; he tells us, point blank (p. 31), speaking of India, that "when cholera is once established in a marching regiment, it continues its course in spite of change of position, food, or other circumstances!" Never did a medical man make an assertion more unpardonable, especially if he applies the term *marching regiment* as it is usually applied. Dr. Hawkins leads us to suppose that he has examined the India reports on cholera. What then are we to think when we find in that for Bengal the following most interesting and conclusive statements ever placed on record? Respecting the Grand Army under the Marquis of Hastings, consisting of 11,500 fighting men, and encamped in November 1817 on the banks of the Sinde, the official report states that the disease "as it were in an instant gained fresh vigour, and at once burst forth with irresistible violence in every direction. Unsubjected to the laws of contact, and proximity of situation, which had been observed to mark and retard the course of other pestilences, it surpassed the plague in the width of its range, and outstripped the most fatal diseases hitherto known, in the destructive rapidity of its progress. Previously to the 14th it had overspread every part of the camp, sparing neither sex nor age, in the undistinguishing virulence of its attacks."—"From the 14th to the 20th or 22d, the mortality had become so general as to depress the stoutest spirits. The sick were already so numerous, and still pouring in so quickly from every quarter, that the medical men, although night and day at their posts, were no longer able to administer to their necessities. The whole camp then put on the appearance of a hospital. The noise and bustle almost inseparable from the intercourse of large bodies of people had nearly subsided. Nothing was to be seen but individuals anxiously hurrying from one division of a camp to another, to inquire after the fate of their dead or dying companions, and melancholy groups of natives bearing the biers of their departed relatives to the river. At length even this consolation was denied to them, for the mortality latterly became so great that there was neither time nor hands to carry off the bodies, which were then thrown into the neighbouring ravines, or hastily committed to the earth on the spots on which they had expired." Let us now inquire how this appalling mortality was arrested;—the report goes on to inform us:—"It was clear that such a frightful state of things could not last long, and that unless some immediate check were given to the disorder, it must soon depopulate the camp. It was therefore wisely determined by the Commander-in-chief *to move in search of a healthier soil and of purer air*," which they found when they "crossed the clear stream of the Bitwah, and upon its high and dry banks at Erich soon got rid of the pestilence, and met with returning health." Now just fancy epidemic cholera a disease transmissible by "susceptible articles," and what an inexhaustible stock must this large army, with its thousands of followers, have long carried about with them; but, instead of this, they were soon in a condition to take the field. Against the above historical fact men of ingenuity may advance what they please. There is no doubt that, in the above instance, severe cases of cholera occurred *during the move*, the poison taken into the system on the inauspicious spot, not having produced its effects at once; it is needless to point out what occurs in this respect in remittent and intermittent fevers. The India reports furnish further evidence of mere removal producing health, where cholera had previously

- 33 -

existed. Mr. Bell, a gentleman who had served in India, and who has lately written upon the disease,[9] informs us (p. 84), that "removing a camp a few miles, has frequently put an entire and immediate stop to the occurrence of new cases; and when the disease prevailed destructively in a village, the natives often got rid of it by deserting their houses for a time, though in doing so they necessarily exposed themselves to many discomforts, which, *cæteris paribus*, we should be inclined to consider exciting causes of an infectious or contagious epidemic." We even find that troops have, as it may be said, *out-marched* the disease, or rather the cause of the disease; that is, moved with rapidity over an extensive surface where the atmosphere was impure, and thereby escaped—on the principle that travellers are in the habit of passing as quickly as they can across the pontine marshes. Mr. Bell says, "In July, 1819, I marched from Madras in medical charge of a large party of young officers who had just arrived in India, and who were on their way to join regiments in the interior of the country. There was also a detachment of Sepoys, and the usual number of attendants and camp-followers of such a party in India. The cholera prevailed at Madras when we left it. Until the 5th day's march (fifty miles from Madras) no cases of the disease occurred. On that day several of the party were attacked on the line of march; and, during the next three stages, we continued to have additional cases. Cholera prevailed in the countries through which we were passing. In consultation with the commanding officer of the detachment, it was determined that we should *leave the disease behind us*; and as we were informed that the country beyond the Ghauts was free from it, we marched, without a halt, until we reached the high table land of Mysore. The consequence was, that we left the disease at Vellore eighty-seven miles from Madras, and we had none of it until we had marched seventy miles further (seven stages), when we again found it at one of our appointed places of encampment; but our camp was, in consequence, pushed on a few miles, and only one case, a fatal one, occurred in the detachment; the man was attacked on the line of march. We again left the disease, and were free from it during the next 115 miles of travelling; we then had it during three stages, and found many villages deserted. We once more left it, and reached our journey's end, 260 miles further, without again meeting it. Thus, in a journey of 560 miles, this detachment was exposed to, and left the disease behind it, four different times; and on none of those occasions did a single case occur beyond the tainted spots." What a lesson for Dr. Hawkins! But *for whom* could Dr. Hawkins have written his *curious* book? Hear Mr. Bell in respect to the common error of the disease following high roads and navigable rivers only:—"I have known the disease to prevail for several weeks at a village in the Southern Mahratta country, within a few miles of the principal station of the district, and then leave that division of the country entirely; or, perhaps, cases would occur at some distant point. In travelling on circuit with the Judge of that district, I have found the disease prevailing destructively in a small and secluded village, while no cases were reported from any other part of the district." What is further stated by Mr. Bell will tend to explain why so much delusion has existed with regard to the progress of the disease being remarkably in the direction of lines of commerce, or great intercourse:—"When travelling on circuit, I have found the disease prevailing in a district *before any report had been made of the fact, notwithstanding the most positive orders on the subject*; and I am persuaded, that were any of the instances adduced in support of the statement under consideration strictly inquired into, it would be found that the usual apathy of the natives of India had prevented their noticing the existence of the disease until the fact was brought prominently forward by the presence of Europeans. It should also be brought to mind, that cholera asphyxia is not a new disease to these natives, but seems to be, in many places, almost endemical, whilst it is well known that strangers, in such circumstances, become more obnoxious to the disease than the inhabitants of the country. Moreover, travellers have superadded to the remote cause of the disease, fatigue and road discomforts, which are not trifling in a country where there are neither inns nor carriages." (p. 89.) Cholera only attacks a certain proportion of a population, and is it wonderful that we should hear more of epidemic on high roads, where the population is greatest? High roads too are often along the course of rivers; and is there not some reason for believing, that there is often along the course of rivers, whether navigable or not, certain conditions of the atmosphere unfavourable to health? When Dr. Hawkins stated, as we find at p. 131 he has done, that where the inhabitants of certain hilly ranges in India escaped the disease, "these have been said to have interdicted all intercourse with the people below," he should have quoted some respectable authority, for otherwise, should we unhappily be visited by this disease, the people of our plains may one day wage an unjust war against the sturdy Highlanders or Welsh mountaineers.[10] Little do the discussers of politics dream of the high interest of this part of the cholera question, and little can they conceive the unnecessary afflictions which the doctrine of the contagionists are calculated to bring on the nation. Let no part of the public suppose for a moment that this is a question concerning medical men more than it does them; *all* are *very* deeply concerned, the heads of families more especially so.

[9] This is by far the best work yet published in England on the cholera, but it is to be regretted that the author has not alluded to the works of gentlemen who have a priority of claim to some of the opinions he has published: I think that, in particular, Mr. Orton's book, printed in India, should have been noticed.

[10] Something of this kind would have infallibly taken place, had certain insane proposals lately made respecting the *shutting in* of the people of Sunderland, been carried into effect.

We see that the identity of the European and Indian epidemic cholera is admitted on all sides; we have abundant proof that whatever can be said as to the progress of the disease, its anomalies, &c., in the former country, have been also noted respecting it in the latter; and Dr. Hawkins, when he put forth his book, had most assuredly abundant materials upon which to form a rational opinion. It is by no small effort, therefore, that I can prevent all the respect due to him from evaporating, when he declares, at page 165, that "the disease in India was *probably* communicable from person to person, and that in Europe it has *undeniably* proved so." But Dr. Hawkins is a Fellow of the College of Physicians, and we must not press this point further than to wish others to recollect that he has told us that he drew up his book in haste; and, moreover, that he wished to gratify the *curiosity* of the public. The Riga story about the hemp and the fifteen labourers I shall leave in good hands, the British Consul's at that city, who was required to draw up, for his government, a statement of the progress, &c. of the cholera there, of which the following is an extract:—

"The fact of non-contagion seems determined, as far as a question can be so, which must rest solely upon negative evidence. The strongest possible proof is, the circumstance, that not one of the persons employed in removing the dead bodies (which is done without any precaution) has been taken ill. *The statement of fifteen labourers being attacked, while opening a pack of hemp, is a notorious falsehood.* Some physicians incline to the opinion, that the disease may sometimes be caught by infection, where the habit of body of the individual is predisposed to receive it; the majority of the faculty, however, maintain a contrary doctrine, and the result of the hospital practice is in their favour. There are 78 persons employed in the principal hospital here; of these only two have been attacked, one of whom was an '*Inspecteur de Salle,*' and not in immediate attendance upon the sick. I am assured that the other hospitals offer the same results, but as I cannot obtain equally authentic information respecting them, I confine myself to this statement, on which you may rely. On the other hand, in private families, several instances have occurred where the illness of one individual has been followed by that of others: but, generally, only where the first case has proved fatal, and the survivors have given way to grief and alarm. Mercenary attendants have seldom been attacked, and, as mental agitation is proved to be one of the principal agents in propagating or generating the disease, these isolated cases are attributed to that cause rather than infection.

"It is impossible to trace the origin of the disease to the barks; indeed it had not manifested itself at the place whence they come till after it had broken out here. The nearest point infected was Schowlen (at a distance of 200 wersts), and it appeared simultaneously in three different places at Riga, without touching the interjacent country. The first cases were two stone-masons, working in the Petersburg suburbs, a person in the citadel, and a lady resident in the town. None of these persons had had the slightest communication with the crews of barks, or other strangers, and the quarter inhabited by people of that description was later attacked, though it has ultimately suffered most.

"None of the medical men entertain the slightest doubt of the action of atmospheric influence—so many undeniable instances of the spontaneous generation of the disease having occurred. Half the town has been visited by diarrhœa, and the slightest deviation from the regimen now prescribed (consisting principally in abstinence from acids, fruit, beer, &c.) invariably produces an attack of that nature, and, generally, cholera: fright, and intoxication, produce the same effect.

"Numerous instances could be produced of persons in perfect health, some of whom had not left their rooms since the breaking out of the disease, having been attacked by cholera, almost instantaneously after having imprudently indulged in sour milk, cucumbers, &c. It is a curious circumstance, bearing on this question, that several individuals coming from Riga have died at Wenden, and other parts of Livonia, without a single inhabitant catching the disease; on the other hand, it spreads in Courland, and on the Prussian frontier, notwithstanding every effort to check its progress. The intemperance of the Russians during the holidays has swelled the number of fresh cases, the progressive diminution of which had previously led us to look forward to a speedy termination of the calamity." This is a pretty fair specimen of the *undeniable* manner in which cholera is proved to be contagious in Europe, and we shall, for the present, leave Dr. Hawkins in possession of the full enjoyment of such proofs.

Some attempt was made at Sunderland, to establish that, in the case which I mentioned in my last as having proved fatal there, the disease had been imported from foreign parts, but due inquiry having been made by the collector of the customs, this proved to be unfounded; the man's name was Robert Henry, a pilot:—he died *on the 14th of August.*[11]

[11] In a former letter I alluded to cases of cholera which appeared this year at Port Glasgow; I find that the highly interesting details of those cases have been just published:—*they should be read by everybody who takes the smallest interest in the important questions connected with the cholera.* The London publishers are Whittaker and Co.

Abroad we find that, unhappily, the cholera has made its appearance at Hamburgh; official information to this effect arrived from our Consul at that place, on Tuesday the 11th inst. (October). The absurdity of cordons and quarantines is becoming daily more evident. By accounts from Vienna, dated the 26th September, the Imperial Aulic Council had directed certain lines of cordon to be broken up, seeing, as is stated, that they were inefficacious; and by accounts of the same date, the Emperor had promised his people not to establish cordons between certain states.

We find at the close of a pamphlet on cholera, lately published by Mr. Searle, a gentleman who served in India, and who was in Warsaw during the greater part of the epidemic which prevailed there this year, the following statement:—"I have only to add, that after all I have heard, either in India or in Poland, after all I have read, seen, or thought upon the subject, I arrive at this conclusion, that the disease is not contagious."

In confirmation of the opinion of Mr. Searle, we have now the evidence of the medical commission sent by the French government to Poland. Dr. Londe, President of that commission, arrived in Paris some days ago. He announced to the minister in whose department the quarantine lies, as well as to M. Hèly D'Oissel, President of the Superior Council of Health, that it was proved in Poland, entirely to his satisfaction, as well as to the satisfaction of his five colleagues, that the cholera *is not a contagious disease.*

The Minister of War also sent *four* medical men to Warsaw. Three of them have already declared against contagion; so it may be presumed that the day is not far distant when those true plagues of society, cordons and quarantines against cholera, shall be abolished. Hear the opinion of a medical Journalist in France,—after describing, a few days ago, the quarantine and cordon regulations in force in that country:—"But what effect is to be produced by these extraordinary measures, this immense display of means, and all these obstructions to the intercourse of communities, against a disease not contagious; a disease propagating itself epidemically; and which nothing has hitherto been able to arrest? To increase its ravages a hundred-fold,—to ruin the country, and to make the people revolt against measures which draw down on them misery and death at the same time." What honest man would not *now* wish that in this country the cholera question were placed *in Chancery*; where, I have no doubt, it would be quickly disposed of. I shall merely add, that the ten medical men sent from France to Poland, for the purpose of studying the nature of cholera, have all remained unattacked by the disease.

October 15, 1831.

LETTER V.

It was well and wisely said, that to know any-thing thoroughly, it must be known in all its details; and, to gain the confidence of the public in the belief of non-contagion in cholera, it is in vain that they are informed that certain alleged facts, brought forward industriously by contagionists, are quite groundless, unless proofs are given showing this to be the case. The public must, in short, have those alleged instances of contagion which have gained currency circumstantially disproved, or they will still listen to a doctrine leading to the disorganization of the community wherever it is acted upon. It is solely upon this ground that these letters have any claim to attention. Dr. James Johnson, of London, has, since my last letter, publicly contradicted, with all the bluntness and energy of honest conviction, the statement by Sir Gilbert Blane, Drs. Macmichael, Hawkins, &c., as to the importation of the cholera into the Mauritius by the Topaze frigate; but *evidence* is what people want on these occasions, and, relative to the case in question, probably the public will consider what is to be found in my third and fourth letters, quite conclusive. Having again mentioned the Mauritius, I cannot refrain from expressing my great surprise that Mr. Kennedy, who has lately published on cholera, should give, with the view of showing "the dread and confusion existing at the time," a proclamation by General Darling, while he does not furnish a word about the result of the proceedings instituted by that officer, as detailed in my third letter, relative to the non-contagious nature of the disease, a point of all others the most important to the public. As to accounts regarding the confusion caused by the appearance of epidemic cholera, we have had no lack of them in the public papers during many months past, from quarters nearer home.

Regarding a statement made by Dr. Hawkins in his book on cholera, viz. "That Moreau de Jonnés has taken great pains to prove that the disease was imported into the Russian province of Orenburg," Dr. H. omits to tell us how completely he failed in the endeavour. In the *Edinburgh Medical and Surgical Journal* for July, 1831, there is a review of a memoir by Professor Lichtenstädt, of St. Petersburg, in which M. Moreau's speculations are put to flight. From the efforts of this *pains-taking* gentleman (M. Moreau) in the cause of contagion in cholera, as well as yellow-fever, he seems to be considered in this country as a medical man; but this is not the case: he raised himself by merit, not only to military rank, but also to literary distinction, and is a member of the Academy of Sciences, where he displays an imagination the most vivid, but as to the sober tact necessary for the investigation of such questions as those connected with the contagion or non-contagion of cholera and yellow-fever, he is considered *below par*. He saw the yellow-fever in 1802-3, at Martinique, while *aid-de-camp* to the Governor, and still adheres to the errors respecting it which he imbibed in his youth, and when he was misled by occurrences taking place *within a malaria boundary*, where hundreds of instances are always at hand, furnishing the sort of *post hoc propter hoc* evidence of contagion with which some people are satisfied, but which is not one bit less absurd, than if a good lady, living in the marshes of Kent, were to insist upon it, that her daughter Eliza took the ague from her daughter Jane, because they lived together. Strange to say, however, M. Casimir Perier, the Prime Minister of France, seems to be guided, according to French journals, by the opinions of this gentleman on cholera, instead of by different medical commissions sent to Warsaw, &c.

The question of contagion in cholera has been now put to the test in every possible way, let us view it for a moment, as compared with what has occurred in regard to typhus at the London Fever Hospital, according to that excellent observer Dr. Tweedie, physician to the establishment. Doubts, as we all know, have been of late years raised as to the contagion of typhus, but I believe nothing that has as yet appeared is so well calculated to remove those doubts as the statements by this gentleman (*see "Illustrations of Fever"*), where he shows that it has been remarked for a series of years that "the resident medical officers, matrons, porters, laundresses, and domestic servants not connected with the wards, and every female who has ever performed the duties of a nurse, have one and all been the subjects of fever,"—while, *in the Small-Pox Hospital*, which adjoins it, according to the statements of the physician, "no case of genuine fever has occurred among the medical officers or domestics of that institution for the last eight years." Had typhus been produced in the attendants by *malaria* of the locality, those persons in the service of the neighbouring Small-Pox Hospital should also have been attacked to a greater or less extent, it is reasonable to suppose, within the period mentioned. Now let this be compared with all that has been stated respecting attendants on cholera patients, and let it be compared with the following excellent fact in illustration, showing how numbers labouring under the disease, and brought from the inauspicious spot where they were attacked to a place occupied by healthy troops, did not, *even under the disadvantage of a confined space*, communicate the disease to a single individual:—"It has been remarked by many practitioners, that although they had brought cholera patients into crowded wards of hospitals, no case of the disease occurred among the sick previously in hospital, or among the hospital attendants. My own experience enables me fully to confirm this. The Military Hospital at Dharwar, an oblong apartment of about 90 feet by 20, was within the fort, and the lines of the garrison were about a mile distant outside of the walls of the fort. On two different occasions (in 1820 and 1821), when the disease prevailed epidemically among the troops of that station, while I was in medical charge of the garrison, but while no cases had occurred in the fort within which the hospital was situated, the patients were brought at once from their quarters to the hospital, which, on each occasion, was crowded with sick labouring under other disorders. No attempt was made to separate the cholera patients. On one of these occasions, no case of cholera occurred within the hospital; on the other, one of the sick was attacked, but he was a convalescent sepoy, who had not been prevented from leaving the fort during the day. The disease, on each of those occasions, was confined to a particular subdivision of the lines, and none of those within the fort were attacked." (*Bell on Cholera*, p. 92.)

I have already quoted from Dr. Zoubkoff of Moscow, once a believer in contagion; every word in his pamphlet is precious; let but the following be read, and who will then say that "the seclusion of the sick should be insisted on?"—"The individuals of the hospitals, including soldiers and attendants on the sick, were about thirty-two in number, who, excepting the medical men, had never attended any sick; we all handled, more or less, the bodies of the patients, the corpses, and the clothes of the sick; have had our hands covered with their cold sweat, and steeped in the bath while the patients were in it; have inhaled their breath and the vapours of their baths; have tasted the drinks contained in their vessels, all without taking any kind of precaution, and all without having suffered any ill effects. We received into our hospital sixty-five cholera patients, and I appeal to the testimony of the thirty-six survivors, whether we took any precautions in putting them into the bath or in handling them—whether we were not seated sometimes on the bed of one, sometimes on that of another, talking to them. On returning home directly from the hospital, and without using chloride of lime, or changing my clothes, I sat down to table with my family, and received the caresses of my children, firmly convinced that I did not bring them a fatal poison either in my clothes or in my breath. Nobody shut his door either against me or my colleagues; nobody was afraid to touch the hand of the physician who came direct from an hospital—that hand which had just before wiped the perspiration from the brow of cholera patients. From the time that people had experience of the disease, nobody that I am aware of shunned the sick." Who, after this, can read over with common patience directions for the separation of a cholera patient from his friends, as if "*an accursed thing?*" or who (*il faut trancher le mot*) will now follow those directions?

As to the good Sir Gilbert Blane, who has distributed far and wide a circular containing a description the most *naïve* on record, of the epidemic cholera, hard must be the heart which could refuse making the allowance which he claims for himself and his memoir; and though he brands those who see, in his account of the marchings and counter-marchings of the disease, nothing on a level with the intellect of the present age, as a parcel of prejudiced imbeciles, we must still feel towards him all the respect due to a parent arrived at a time of life when things are not as they were wont to be, *nec mens, nec ætas.* I may be among those he accuses of sometimes employing "unintelligible jargon," but shall not retort while I confess my inability to understand such expressions as "some obscure occurrence of unwholesome circumstances" which seem to have, according to him, both "brought" the disease to Jessore in 1817, and produced it there at the same time. Sir Gilbert marks out for the public what he considers as forming one of the principal differences between the English and Indian cholera, viz. that in the latter the discharges "consist of a liquid resembling thin gruel, in the English disease they are feculent and bilious." Now if he has read the India reports, he must have found abundance of evidence showing that sometimes there were *even bilious stools*[12] not at all like what he describes; and, again, if he is in the habit of reading the journals, he must have found *abundant* evidence of malignant cholera with discharges like water-gruel in this country. As to the French Consul at Aleppo having escaped with 200 other individuals confined to his residence, I shall only say, as it is Sir Gilbert Blane who relates the circumstance, that he *forgot* to mention that the aforesaid persons had retired to a residence *outside* the city; which, permits me to assure you, Sir Gilbert, just makes all the difference in hundreds of cases:—they happened to retire to "*clene air,*" and had they carried 50 ague cases or 50 cholera cases with them (it matters not one atom which), the result would have been exactly the same. The mention of Barcelona and the yellow-fever, by Sir Gilbert, was, as Dr. Macmichael would term it, rather *unlucky* for his cause, though probably lucky for humanity; for it cannot be too generally known that, during the yellow-fever epidemic there in 1821, more than 60,000 people left the city, and spread themselves all over Spain, without a single instance of the disease having been communicated, WHILE, AT BARCELONETTA, THE INFAMOUS CORDON SYSTEM PREVENTED THE UNFORTUNATE INHABITANTS FROM GOING BEYOND THE WALLS, AND THE CONSEQUENCES OF SHUTTING THEM UP WERE MOST HORRID.

[12] See Orton on Cholera, who is most explicit upon this point, and cites from the India Reports:—so that the distinctions attempted to be drawn in this respect between the "cholera of India," and that of other countries, are, after all, *quite untenable.*

Little need be said respecting the pure assumptions of Sir Gilbert as to the movements of the malady by land and by water, for those vague and hacknied statements have been again and again refuted; but we may remark that whereas all former accounts respecting the cholera in 1817, in the army of the Marquis of Hastings, state that the disease broke out somewhat suddenly in the camp on the banks of the Sinde, Sir Gilbert, without deigning to give his authority, makes the army set out for "Upper India accompanied by this epidemic." We find that Mr. Kennedy, another advocate for contagion in cholera, differs from Sir Gilbert as to the disease having accompanied the grand army on the march; for he says the appearance of the malady was announced in camp in the early part of November, when "the first cases excited little alarm." In referring, in a former letter, to the sickness in the above army, I showed from the text of the Bengal report, how a change of position produced a return of health in the troops; but Mr. Kennedy states that the disease had greatly declined a few days before the removal, so that it had lost "its infecting power." Nevertheless it appears by this gentleman's account, a little farther on, that "in their progressive movement the grounds which they occupied during the night as temporary encampments were generally found in the morning, strewed with the dead like a field of battle"! This gentleman tells us that he has laid down a law of "increase and decline appertaining to cholera," by which, and the assistance of *currents of contagion*, it would appear all these things are reconciled wonderfully. Several of the points upon which he grounds his belief of contagion have been already touched upon in these letters, and the rest, considering the state of the cholera question in Europe just now, may be allowed to pass at whatever value the public may, after due examination, think it is entitled to. Let it be borne in mind that all contagionists who speak of the cholera in the army of the Marquis of Hastings, forget to tell us that though many thousand native followers had fled from that army during the epidemic, the disease did not appear in the towns situated in the surrounding country, *till the following year*, as may be seen at a glance by reference to Mr. Kennedy's and other maps.

We have another contagionist in the field—a writer in the *Foreign Quarterly Review*, the value of whose observations may appear from his statement, that "in 1828 the disease broke out in Orenburg, and was supposed [*supposed!*] to have been introduced by the caravans which arrive there from Upper Asia, or [*or*, nothing like a second string] by the Kingiss-Cossacks, who are adjoining this town, and were said [*were said!*] to have been about this time affected with the disease." This single extract furnishes an excellent specimen of the sort of *proofs* which the contagionists, to a man, seem to be satisfied with as to the cholera being "carried" from place to place. This gentleman must surely be under some very erroneous impression, when he states that, "According to the reports of the Medical Board of Ceylon, the disease made its appearance in 1819 at Jaffnah in Ceylon, imported from Palamcottah, with which Jaffnah holds constant intercourse, and thence it was propagated over the island." Now there is every reason to believe that a reference to the documents from Ceylon will shew that no report as to the importation of the disease was ever drawn up, for Drs. Farrel and Davy, as well as Messrs. Marshall, Nicholson, and others, who served in that island, are, to this hour, clearly against contagion. But as the writer tells us that he is furnished with unpublished documents respecting the cholera at St. Petersburg, by the chief of the medical department of the quarantine in this country, we do not think it necessary to say one word more—*ex pede Herculem.*

I rejoice to observe that Dr. James Johnson has, at last, *spoken out* upon the quarantine question; and I trust that others will now follow his example. It is only to be regretted, that a gentleman possessing such influence with the public as Dr. Johnson does, should have so long with-held his powerful aid on the occasion; but his motives were, I am quite sure, most conscientious; and I believe that he, as well as others, might have been prevented by a feeling of delicacy from going beyond a certain point.

Since my last letter a code of regulations, in the anticipation of cholera, has been published by the Board of Health. *Let our prayers be offered up with fervency tenfold greater than before, that our land may not be afflicted with this dire malady.* The following statement, however, may not be altogether useless at this moment. According to the *Journal des Debats* of the 24th instant, the Emperor of Austria, in a letter to his High Chancellor, dated Schœnbrunn, October 10th, and published in the *Austrian Observer* of the 12th, formally makes the most magnanimous declaration to his people, THAT HE HAD COMMITTED AN ERROR IN ADOPTING THE VEXATIOUS AND WORSE-THAN USELESS QUARANTINE AND CORDON REGULATIONS AGAINST CHOLERA; that he did so before the nature of the disease was so fully understood; admits that those regulations have been found, after full experience, to have produced consequences more calamitous than those arising from the disease itself ("*plus funeste encore que les maux que provenaient de la maladie elle-même.*") He kindly makes excuses for still maintaining a modified quarantine system at certain points, in consequence, as he states, of the opinions still existing in the dominions of some of his neighbours, *for otherwise his commercial relations would be broken off. To secure his maritime intercourse, he must do as they do!* We find that as *all* the Prussian cordons have been dissolved, *their vessels* are excluded from entrance into certain places on the Elbe. What a horrid state of things! But, as a reference will shew, this was one of the things stated in my first letter as likely to occur: it is surely a fit subject for immediate arrangement between governments. In the mean time, we cannot but profit by the great lesson just received from Austria.

I shall add no more on the present occasion, than that my last information from Edinburgh notifies the death, from *Scotch cholera*, of two respectable females in that city, after an illness of only a few hours.

LETTER VI.

At a moment when the subject of cholera has become so deeply interesting, the good of the public can surely not be better consulted by the press than when it devotes its columns (even to the exclusion of some political and other questions of importance) to details of plain facts connected with the contagious or non-contagious nature of that malady—a *question beyond all others regarding it, of most importance,* for upon it must hinge all sanatory or conservative regulations, and a mistake must, in the event of an epidemic breaking out, directly involve thousands in ruin. In the case of felony, where but the life of a single individual is at stake—nay, not only in the case of felony, but in the case of a simple misdemeanour, or even in the simple case of debt—we see the questions of yes or no examined by the Judges of the land with due rigour; while, on the point to which I refer, and which affects so deeply the dearest interests of whole communities, evidence has been acted upon so vague as to make some people fancy that we have retrograded to the age of witchcraft. Be it recollected that we shall not have the same excuse as some of our continental neighbours had for running into frightful errors—for we have their dear-bought experience laid broadly before us; and to profit duly by it, it only requires a scrutiny by a tribunal, wholly, if you please, non-medical, such as may be formed within an hour in this metropolis; nothing short of this will do. All, till then, will be vacillation; and when the enemy does come in force, we shall find ourselves just as much at a loss how to act as our continental neighbours were on the first appearance of cholera among them; I say after its first appearance, for we find that they all discovered, plainly enough latterly, what was best to be done. Small indeed may be the chance of the present order of things as to quarantines, the separation of persons attacked, &c., being changed by anything which I can offer; but, having many years experience of disease—having had no small share of experience in this disease in particular, and having, perhaps, paid as much attention to all that has been said about it as any man living, I should be wanting in my duty towards God and man did I not protest, most loudly, against those regulations, which shall have for their base, an assumption, that a being affected with cholera can, IN ANY MANNER WHATEVER, transmit, or communicate, the disease to others, *however close or long continued the intercourse may be*; because such doctrine is totally in opposition to all the fair or solid evidence now before the public;—because it is calculated, in numberless instances, to predispose the constitution to the disease, by exciting terror equal to that in the case of plague;—because it is teaching us Christians to do what Jews, and others, never do, to abandon the being who has so many

- 45 -

ties upon our affections;—because the desertion of friends and relatives, and the being left solely in charge, perhaps, of a feeble and aged hireling (if even such can be got, which I much doubt when terror is so held out,) must tend directly to depress those functions which, from the nature of the disease, it should be our great effort to support;—finally, because a proper and unbiassed examination of the question will shew, that all these horrors are likely to arise out of regulations which may, with equal justice, be applied to ague, to the remittent fevers of some countries, or to the Devonshire cholic, as to cholera.

Happily, it is not yet too late to set about correcting erroneous opinions, pregnant with overwhelming mischief, for hitherto the measures acted upon have only affected our commerce and finances to a certain extent; but it appears to me that not a moment should be lost, in order to prevent a public panic; and, in order to prevent those calamities which, in addition to the effects of the disease itself, occurred, as we have seen, on the Continent. Let then, I say, a Commission be forthwith appointed, composed of persons accustomed to weigh evidence in other cases, and who will not be likely to give more than its due weight to the authority of any individuals. Let this be done, and, in the decision, we shall be sure to obtain all that human wisdom can arrive at on so important a subject; and the public cannot hesitate to submit to whatever may afterwards be proposed. It will then be seen whether the London Board of Health have decided as wisely as they have hastily. For my part, I shall for ever reject what may be held as evidence in human affairs, if it be not shewn that an individual attending another labouring under cholera, runs no further risk of being infected than an individual attending an ague patient does of being infected by this latter disease. What a blessing (in case of our being visited by an epidemic) should this turn out to be the decision of those whose opinions would be more likely to be regarded by the public than mine are likely to be.

Many, I am quite aware, are the professional men of experience now in this country, who feel with me on this occasion, but who, in deference to views emanating from authority, refrain from coming forward:—let me entreat them, however, to consider the importance of their suggestions to the community at large, at this moment; and let me beg of them to come forward and implore government to institute a special commission for the re-consideration of measures, founded on evidence the most vague that it is possible to conceive; or, perhaps, I should rather say, *against* whatever deserves the name of evidence. Every feeling should be sacrificed, by professional men, for the public good; we must even run the greatest risk of incurring the displeasure of those of our friends who are in the Board of Health. That we do run some risk is pretty plain, from the conduct of a vile journalist closely connected with an individual of a paid party, who has threatened us unbelievers in generally-exploded doctrines, with a fate nothing short of that which overwhelmed some of the inhabitants of Pompeii.

Let me ask why *all* the documents of importance forwarded to the Board of Health are not published in the collection just issued? Why are those forwarded by *the Medical Gentleman sent to Dantzic* not published.[13] Why has not an important document forwarded by our Consul at Riga not been published? Above all, why has not allusion been made in their papers to those cases of PURE SPASMODIC CHOLERA, which have occurred in various parts of England within the last five months, and the details of which has been faithfully transmitted to them. If those cases be inquired into thoroughly and impartially, and that several of them be not found to be PERFECTLY IDENTIC with the epidemic cholera of India, of Russia, &c., I hereby promise the public to disclose my name, and to suffer all the ignomy of a person making false statements. Indeed, I may confidently assure the public, that in at least one case which occurred about two months ago, the opinion of a gentleman who had practiced in India, and who had investigated the history of the symptoms, the identity with those of Asiatic cholera, was not denied. The establishment of this point is of itself sufficient to overthrow all supposition as to the importation of the disease.

[13] Since the above was written, I find that this gentleman has adduced the strongest proofs possible against contagion.

In the case of Richard Martin, whose death occurred at Sunderland about two months ago—in the case of Martin M'Neal, of the 7th Fusileers, which occurred at Hull, on the 11th of August last—in the cases at Port Glasgow, as detailed in a pamphlet by Dr. Marshall of that place—as well as several other cases which occurred throughout the year, and the details of many of which are in possession of the Board of Health—the advocates, *"par metier,"* of contagion in cholera, have not a loop-hole to creep out at. Take but a few of the symptoms in one of those cases as taken down by the Medical Gentleman in charge,—"The body was cold, and covered by a clammy sweat—the features completely sunk—*the lips blue*, the face discoloured—tongue moist and very cold—the hands and feet blue, cold, and as if steeped in water, like a washerwoman's hand; the extremities cold to the axillæ and groins, and no pulse discoverable lower; the voice changed, and the speech short and laborious. He answered with reluctance, and in monosyllables." This man had the pale dejections, and several other symptoms, considered so characteristic of the Asiatic cholera; yet no spreading took place from him, nor ever will in similar cases. With the exception of the vomiting and purging, there is, in the state of patients labouring under this form of cholera, a great similarity to the first stage of the malignant fevers of the Pontine Marshes, and many other places, and the patient need not be one bit the more avoided. Let this be, therefore, no small consolation, when we find that, by the official news of this day, five more deaths have occurred at Sunderland.

Nov. 9, 1831.

LETTER VII.

It may be inferred, from what I have stated at the close of my letter of yesterday, that if a Commission be appointed, I look forward to its being shewn, as clear as the sun at noon day, that the most complete illusion has existed, and, on the part of many, still exists, with regard to the term *Indian* or *Asiatic* cholera; for a form of cholera possessing characters quite peculiar to the disease in that country, and unknown, till very lately, in other countries, *has never existed there.* Cholera, from a cause as inscrutable, perhaps, as the cause of life itself, has prevailed there, and in other parts of the world, in its severest forms, and to a greater extent than previously recorded; but, whether we speak of the mild form, or of a severe form, proceeding or not to the destruction of life, the symptoms have everywhere been precisely the same. In this country it has been over and over again remarked, that, so far back as 1669, the spasmodic cholera prevailed epidemically under the observation of Dr. Sydenham, who records it. For many years after the time of Dr. Cullen, who frequently promulgated opinions founded on those of some fancy author rather than on his own observation, it was very much the fashion to speak of redundancy of bile, or of acrid bile, as the cause of the whole train of symptoms in this disease; but, since the attention of medical men has been more particularly drawn to the subject, practitioners may be found in every town in England who can inform you that, in severe cases of cholera, they have generally observed that no bile whatever has appeared till the patient began to get better. Abundance of cases of this kind are furnished by the different medical journals of this year. In fifty-two cases of cholera which passed under my observation in the year 1828, the *absence* of bile was always most remarkable. I made my observations with extraordinary care. One of the cases proved fatal, in which the group of symptoms deemed characteristic of the Indian or Indo-Russian cholera, was most perfect, and in the mass, the symptoms were as aggravated as they have often been observed to be in India;—in several, spasms, coldness of the body, and even convulsions, having been present.

To those who have attended to the subject of cholera, nothing can be more absurd than to hear people say such or such a case cannot be *the true* cholera, or the Indian cholera, or the Russian cholera, because *all* the symptoms ever mentioned are not present: as if, in the epidemic cholera of India and other places, even some of the symptoms considered the most prominent (as spasms, and the disturbance of the stomach and bowels) were not often absent, and that too in some of the most rapidly, fatal cases!

I feel persuaded that much injustice is done to a gentleman lately sent to Sunderland, in attributing to him the very ridiculous opinion, *that because* the disease did not spread, it was *therefore* not identical with the Indian cholera. No person is justified in speaking of the cholera of India as a disease *sui gineris*, and in which a certain group of severe symptoms are always present, when evidence, such as the following is on record:—"On the 22nd instant, when the men had been duly warned of their danger from not reporting themselves sooner, I got into hospital a different description of cases, viz.—men with a full pulse, hot skin," &c. (*Dr. Burrell to Dr. Milne, Seroor, 27th of July, 1818*)—"But I must tell you that we have, too, cases of common cholera." (*Mr. Craw, Seroor—Bengal Report, p. 48*)—"The cases which terminated favourably presented very different symptoms [from the low form of the disease.] As I saw the men immediately after they were attacked, they came to me with a quick *full* pulse, and in several instances pain in the head; there was no sweating."—"in several cases *bile* appeared from the first in considerable quantities in the egesta; and these were more manageable than those in which no bile was ejected, although the spasms and vomiting (the most distressing symptoms of the complaint) were equally violent." (*Mr. Campbell, Seroor,—see Orton, 2nd ed. p. 18*)—"In conclusion, I am happy to inform you that, for the last three days the disease has been evidently on the decline, and, during that period, most of the cases have assumed a different and much milder type, and, comparatively, are little dangerous. It approaches somewhat to fever; the patient complains of severe pain in the legs, sometimes vomiting a watery fluid, and sometimes bile." (*White—Bengal Reports, p. 68.*)

The same gentleman afterwards observes, "The disease continues to present a milder aspect, and now occurs but rarely: loss of pulse and coldness are seldom observed."

On the decline of a particular epidemic, Mr. Alardyce observed many cases in the 34th regiment, with *bilious* discharges throughout. (Orton, 1st Ed. 128). Finally, referring to the work of Mr. Orton, a gentleman who served in India, and who, being a contagionist, will be considered, I suppose, not bad authority by those who are of his opinion, we find the following declaration. (p. 26, 1st Ed.) "My own experience has been very conclusive with regard to the sthenic form of the disease. I have found a very considerable number of cases exhibiting, singly, or in partial combination, every possible degree, and almost every kind of increased action."—"Very full, hard, and quick pulse, hot skin, and flushed surface; evacuations of bile, [you are requested to note this, reader] both by vomiting and stool, from the commencement of the attack. And, finally, I have seen some of those cases passing into the low form of the disease."—"The inference from these facts is plain, however opposite these two forms of disease may appear, *there is no essential or general difference between them.*" After such authorities, and what has elsewhere been shewn, can any cavelling be for one moment permitted as to the cholera in Sunderland not being of the same nature as that of India? It may be now clearly seen that in India as in Sunderland, the same variety of grades occurred in the disease.

In making my communications for the benefit of the public, it is my wish to spare the feelings of Sir Gilbert Blane; but as he persists in giving as facts often refuted tales of contagion, in order to uphold doctrines which he must observe are tumbling into ruins in all directions, it becomes necessary that his work of mischief should no longer remain unnoticed.

Not a single circumstance which he quotes relative to the marchings and the voyages of the contagion of cholera will bear the slightest examination; and yet he has detailed them as if, on his simple assertion, they were to be received as things proved, and, consequently, as so many points to be held in view when the public are in search of rules whereby they may be guided. The examination of his assumed facts for one short hour, by a competent tribunal, would prove this to be the case; here it is impossible to enter upon them all: but let us just refer to his *management* of the question relative to the importation of the disease into the Mauritius by the *Topaze* frigate, which he says was not believed there to be the case—and *why* was it not believed? Sir Gilbert takes special care not to tell the public, but they now have the reason from me, at page 22.

If a commission be appointed, half an hour will suffice to place before them, from the medical office in Berkeley-street, the reports alluded to from the Mauritius, by which it is made apparent that long before the arrival of the aforesaid frigate, the disease had shown itself in the Mauritius.[14] What is the public to think of us and our profession, when vague statements are daily attempted to be passed as facts, by contagionists *enragés*? One more short reference to Sir Gilbert's facts.—While referring to the progress of cholera in India, &c. from 1817, he says, in a note, "it is remarkable enough that while the great oriental epidemic appeared thus on the eastern extremity of the Mediterranean, the great western pestilence, the yellow fever, was raging in its western extremity, Gibraltar, Malaga, Barcelona, Leghorn, &c." Now, it is a historical fact, that, at Gibraltar, this disease did not appear between 1814 and 1828—*and at Leghorn not since 1804!* At Malaga, I believe, it did not prevail since 1814! So we have here a pretty good specimen of the accuracy of some of those who undertake to come forward as guides to the public on an occasion of great urgency and peril. By some of Sir Gilbert's abettors, we are assured that his "facts are perfectly reconcileable with the hypothesis of the cholera being of an infectious nature." A fig for all hypothesis just now! Let us have something like the old English trial by jury. May I be allowed to introduce a fresh evidence to the public notice, in addition to the thousand-and-one whose testimony is already recorded. He is worthy of belief for two good reasons in particular; the one because he still (unable to explain what can never be explained, perhaps), calls himself a contagionist, and, in the next place, the statements being from a high official personage, he could not offer them unless true to his Government, as hundreds might have it in their power to contradict them if not accurate. My witness is not a Doctor, but a *Duke*—the Duke de *Mortemar*, lately Ambassador from the French Court to St. Petersburg, who has just published a pamphlet on cholera, a few short extracts from which, but those most important ones, I shall here give. Read them!—people of all classes, read them over and over again! "An important truth seems to be proved by what we shall here relate, which is, that woods seem to diminish the influence of cholera, and that cantons in the middle of thick woods, and placed in the centre of infected countries, have altogether escaped the devastating calamity!"—"The island of Kristofsky, placed in the centre of the populous islands of St. Petersburg, communicating with each other by two magnificent bridges, and with the city by thousands of boats, which carried every day, and particularly on Sundays, a great number of people to this charming spot. The island of Kristofsky, we say, *was preserved completely from attacks of the cholera*; there was not a *single* person ill of the disease in three villages upon it." He continues to state particulars, which, for want of time, cannot be here given, and adds—"To what is this salubrity of Kristofsky, inhabited by the same sort of people as St. Petersburg, to be attributed, fed in the same manner, and following a similar *regime*,—communicating with each other daily, if it be not to the influence of the superb forest which shelters it? The firs, which are magnificent as well as abundant, surround the houses."[15] He notices that the town is low and humid, and that "it is made filthy every Sunday by the great numbers who resort to it, and who gorge themselves with intoxicating drink." In a third letter I shall be able to furnish further extracts from this most interesting pamphlet.

[14] I am aware that very lately certain memoranda have been referred to from the surgeon, but this is merely an expiring effort, and of no avail against the official Report drawn up.

[15] As these most remarkable circumstances have not appeared in the statements of our Russian medical commission, we must either presume that the Duke is not correct, or that those facts have *escaped the notice* of the commission.

In a letter lately inserted in a newspaper, the greatest injustice is done to the Board of Health by the comments made on their recommendations for the *treatment* of cholera—*it is not true* that they have reccommended *specifics*, and I must add my feeble voice in full approbation of all they have suggested on this point. Let the public remark that they most judiciously point at the application of *dry* heat, not baths, which always greatly distress the patient, and, indeed, have sometimes been observed (that is, where the coldness and debility are very great) to accelerate a fatal issue. Of all the arrangements to which a humane public can direct their attention, there is nothing so essential as warmth. I would, therefore, humbly beg to suggest, that funds for the purpose of purchasing coals for gratuitous issue to the poor should be at once established in all directions. Too much, I think, has been said about ventilation and washing, and too little about this.

November 10th.

LETTER VIII.

Already has the problem of the contagious or non-contagious nature of this disease been solved upon our own land; and as sophistry can no longer erect impediments to the due distribution of the resources of this pre-eminently humane nation, it is to be hoped that not an hour will be lost in shaping the arrangements accordingly. What now becomes of the doctrine of a poison, piercing and rapid as the sun's rays, emanating from the bodies of the sick—nay, from the bodies of those who are not sick, but who have been near them or near their houses? In the occurrences at Newcastle and Sunderland, how has the fifty times refuted doctrine of the disease spreading from a point in *two* ways, or in one way, tallied with the facts? We were desired to believe that in India, Persia, &c., "the contagion *travelled*," as the expression is, very slow, because this entity of men's brains was obliged to wend its way with the march of a regiment, or with the slow caravan: now, however, when fifty facilities for the most rapid conveyance have been afforded every hour since its first appearance, it will not put itself one bit out of its usual course. And then what dangers to the attendants on the sick to the members of the same family—to the washerwomen—to the clergymen—to the buriers of the dead—even to those who passed the door of the poor sufferer! Well, what of all this has occurred? Why it has occurred that this doctrine, supported by many who were honest, but had not duly examined alleged facts, and by others, I regret to say, whose interests guided their statements—that the absurdity of this doctrine has now been displayed in the broad light of day. Make allowance (even in this year of great notoriety for susceptibility to cholera in the people at large in this country) for *insusceptibility* on the part of numbers who came into contact at Sunderland and Newcastle, with the persons of cholera patients, with their beds, their furniture, their clothes, &c., yet, if there had ever been the slightest foundation for the assertions of the contagionists, what numbers *ought* to have been contaminated, in all directions over the face of the country, even within the first few days, considering the wonderful degree of intercourse kept up between all parts. But we find that, as in Austria and Prussia, "*la maladie de la terre*" is not disposed here to accommodate itself to vain speculations. *Now* the matter may be reduced to the simple rules of arithmetic, viz.:—if, as "contagionists *par metier*" say, the poison from the body of one individual be, in the twinkling of an eye, and in more ways than one, transmitted to the bodies of a certain number who have been near him, &c., how many thousands, or tens of thousands, in every direction, should, in a multiplied series of communications and transmissions, be now affected?

Those who have watched the course of matters connected with cholera in this country, have not failed to perceive, for some time past, the intent and purport of the assertion so industriously put forth—that the disease might be introduced by people in perfect health; and we have just seen how this *ruse* has been attempted to be played off at Sunderland, as the history of such matters informs us has been done before in other instances, and public vengeance invoked most *foully and unjustly* upon the heads of guiltless persons in the Custom House or Quarantine Department, for "permitting a breach of regulations;" but the several pure cases of spasmodic cholera, in many parts of England besides Sunderland, long before—months before—the arrival of *the* ship (as shewn in a former letter) leave no pretence for any supposition of this kind.

I request that the public may particularly remark, that, frequently as those cases have been cited as proofs of the absurdity of *expecting the arrival* of the disease by a ship, THEIR IDENTITY HAS NEVER ONCE BEEN DISPUTED BY THOSE MOST ANXIOUS TO PROVE THEIR CASE. No; the point has, in common parlance, been always *shirked*; for whoever should doubt it, would only hold himself up to the ridicule of the profession, and to admit it would be to give up the importation farce.

Others have remarked before me that, though a very common, it is a very erroneous mode of expression, to say of cholera, that *it has travelled* to such or such a place, *or has arrived* at such or such places, for it is *the cause* of the malady which is found to prevail, for a longer or shorter time, at those different points. It cannot be expected that people should explain such matters, for, with regard to them, our knowledge seems to be in its infancy, and "we want a sense for atoms." However, as people's minds are a good deal occupied upon the point, and as many are driven to the idea of contagion in the face even of evidence, from not being able to make any thing of this *casse-tête*, the *best guess* will probably be found in the quotation from Dr. Davy, at page 19.

I perceive that the Berlin Gazette is humanely occupied in recommending others to profit by the mistakes regarding contagion which occurred in that country:—"Dr. Sacks, in No. 38 of his Cholera Journal, published here, has again shewn, against Dr. Rush, the fallibility of the doctrine of contagion, as well as the mischievous impracticability of the attempts founded on it to arrest the progress of the disorder by cutting off the communications. It is to be hoped that the alarm so methodically excited by scientific and magisterial authority in the countries to the west of us [!!] will cease, after the ample experience which we have dearly purchased (with some popular tumults), and that the system of incommunication will be at once done away with by all enlightened governments, after what has passed among us."—I am sure, good people, nobody can yet say whether those calling

- 55 -

themselves scientific, will allow us to profit by your sad experience; but I believe that the people of Sunderland are not to be shut in, but allowed to remove, if they choose, in spite of silly speculations.

It may not be uninteresting to mention here, that there are no quarantines and no choleras in Bohemia or Hanover.

LETTER IX.

The following statement from the Duke de Mortemar will be considered probably, very curious, considering that, as already stated, he seems to believe in something like contagion—and for no earthly reason, one may suppose, than from his inability to satisfy himself of the existence of another cause—as if it were not sufficient to prove that in reality the moon *is not* made of green cheese, but one must prove *what it is* made of! But, to the quotation—"The conviction now established, that intercourse with sick produces no increase of danger, should henceforth diminish the dread of this calamity (the cholera). It differs from the plague in this, that it does not, by its sole appearance, take away all hope of help, and destroy all the ties of family and affection. Henceforth those attacked will not be abandoned without aid and consolation; and separation or removal to hospital, the source of despair, will no longer increase the danger. The sick may in future be attended without fears for one's self, or for those with whom we live." How delightful is the simplicity of truth! Why, Sir, a morceau like this, and from an honourable man, let him call himself contagionist or what he may, is more precious at this moment than Persian turkois or Grecian gems. Make me an example, men say, of the culprits "who let the cholera morbus into Sunderland," concealed in "susceptible" articles!—yes, and that we may be on a level in other matters, destroy me some half dozen witches, too, as we were wont to do of yore. But let us have more tidings from Russia to comfort the country of our affections in the hour of her affliction, when so much craft and subtlety is on foot to scare her. Dr. Lefevre, physician to our embassy at St. Petersburg, has just given to the public an account of his observations there during the epidemic, from which the following extracts are made:—

"As far as my practice is concerned both in the quarter allotted to me, and also in private houses in different parts of the town, I have no proof whatever that the disease is contagious.

"The first patient I saw was upon the third day of the epidemic, and upon strict inquiry I could not trace the least connexion between the patient, or those who were about her person, with that part of the town where it first appeared—a distance of several versts.

"As regards the attendants of the sick, in no one instance have I found them affected by the disease, though in many cases they paid the most assiduous attention, watched day and night by the beds of the afflicted, and administered to all their wants.

"I knew four sisters watch anxiously over a fifth severely attacked with cholera, and yet receive no injury from their care.

"In one case I attended a carpenter in a large room, where there were at least thirty men, who all slept on the floor among the shavings; and, though it was a severe and fatal case, no other instance occurred among his companions.

"In private practice, among those in easy circumstances, I have known the wife attend the husband, the husband the wife, parents their children, children their parents, and in fatal cases, where, from long attendance and anxiety of mind, we might conceive the influence of predisposition to operate, in no instance have I found the disease communicated to the attendants."—p. 32, 33.

"The present disease has borne throughout the character of an epidemic, and when the proofs advanced in proof of its contagion have been minutely examined, they have been generally found incorrect; whereas it is clear and open to every inquirer, that the cholera did not occur in many places which had the greatest intercourse with St. Petersburg at the height of the malady, and that it broke out in many others which have been subjected to the strictest quarantine."—p. 34.[16]

[16] It is remarkable enough that Aretæus, who lived, according to some authors, in the first century, gives exactly the same reason which Dr. Lefevre does for the suppression of urine in cholera. So true it is, that that symptom, considered as one of the characteristics of the Indian cholera, was observed in ancient times.

Hear all this, Legislators! Boards of Health throughout the country, hear it! Then you will be able to judge how exceedingly frivolous the idle *opinions* and *reports* are which you have obtruded so industriously upon your notice.

But one more short quotation from Dr. Lefevre, a gentleman certainly not among the number of those who stand denounced before the professional world as unworthy of belief. He says:—"As for many reports which have been circulated, and which, *primâ facie*, seem to militate against the statement [communication to attendants, &c.]. I have endeavoured to pay the most impartial attention to them; but I have never found, upon thorough investigation, that their correctness could be relied upon: and in many instances I have ascertained them to be designedly false."— DESIGNEDLY FALSE! Alas! *toute ça on trouve dans l'article* HOMME; and any body who chooses to investigate, as I have done, the history of epidemics, will find that falsehoods foul have been resorted to—shamelessly resorted to—by persons having a direct interest in maintaining certain views. Enough, then, has been said to put Boards of Health, &c. on their guard against admitting *facts* for their guidance from any quarter whatever, if the purity of the source be not right well established. There is too much at stake just now to permit of our yielding with ill-timed complaisance to *any authority* without observing this very necessary preliminary.

One word, and with all due respect, before closing, on the subject of Dr. James Johnson's "*contingent* contagion," which, though occurring in some diseases, and extremely *feasible* in regard to others, will, if he goes over the evidence again, I am sure, be shown not to apply to cholera, which is strictly a disease of *places*, not persons, and can no more be generated by individuals than ague itself can. I can only say of it, with the philosophic poet, that—

--------------------"A secret venom oft
Corrupts the air, the water, and the land."

Mr. Searle, an English gentleman, well known for his work on cholera, has just returned from Warsaw, where he had the charge of the principal cholera hospital during the epidemic. The statements of this gentleman respecting contagion, being now published, I am induced from their high interest to give them here:—

"I have only to add my most entire conviction that the disease is not contagious, or, in other words, communicable from one person to another in the ordinary sense of the words—a conviction, which, is founded not only upon the nature of the disease, but also upon observations made with reference to the subject, during a period of no less than fourteen years. Facts, however, being deservedly of more weight than mere opinions, I beg leave to adduce the following, in the hope of relieving the minds of the timid from that groundless alarm, which might otherwise not only interfere with or prevent the proper attendance upon the sick, but becomes itself a pre-disposing or exciting cause of the disease; all parties agreeing that of all the debilitating agencies operating upon the human system, there is no one which tends to render it so peculiarly susceptible of disease, and of cholera in particular, than fear.

"The facts referred to are these:—during two months of the period, that I was physician to the principal hospital at Warsaw, devoted to the reception and treatment of this disease, out of about thirty persons attached to the hospital, the greater number of them were in constant attendance upon the sick, which latter were, to the number of from thirty to sixty, constantly under treatment; there were, therefore, patients in every stage of the disease. Several of these attendants, slept every night in the same apartments with the sick, on the beds which happened to be unoccupied, with all the windows and doors frequently closed. These men, too, were further employed in assisting at the dissection of, and sewing up of, the bodies of such as were examined, which were very numerous; cleansing also the dissecting-room, and burying the dead. And yet, notwithstanding all this, only one, during the period of two months, was attacked by the disease, and this an habitual drunkard, under circumstances, which entirely negative contagion, (supposing it to exist), as he had nothing whatever to do with the persons of the sick, though he occasionally assisted at the interment of the dead. He was merely a subordinate assistant to the apothecary, who occupied a detached building with some of the families of the attendants; all of whom likewise escaped the disease. This man, I repeat, was the only one attacked, and then under the following circumstances."

Here Mr. S. relates how this man, having been intoxicated for several days—was, as a punishment locked up almost naked in a damp room for two nights, having previously been severely beaten.

From the foregoing facts, and others pretty similar in all parts of the world where this disease has prevailed, we are, I think, fairly called upon to discard all special pleading, and to admit that man's *best endeavours* have not been able *to make it* communicable by any manner of means.

LETTER X.

At a meeting held some days ago by the members of the Royal Academy of Medicine of Paris, Dr. Londe (President of the French Medical Commission sent to Poland to investigate the nature of the cholera) stated, with regard to the questions of the origin and *communicability* of the disease, that it appeared by a document to which he referred, that 1st. "The cholera did not exist in the Russian corps which fought at *Iganie*," the place where the first battle with the Poles took place. 2d. "That the two thousand Russian prisoners taken on that occasion, and observed at Praga for ten days under the most perfect separation, [*dans un isolement complet*] did not give a single case of cholera." 3d. "That the corps [of the Polish army] which was not at *Iganie*, had more cases of cholera than those which were there." Dr. Londe stated cases of the spontaneous development of the disease in different individuals—of a French Lady confined to her bed, during two months previous to her attack of cholera, of which she died in twenty-two hours—of a woman of a religious order, who had been confined to her bed for six months, and while crossing a balcony, the aspect of which was to the Vistula, was attacked with cholera, and died within four hours. Dr. Londe, among other proofs that the disease was not transmissible, or, as some prefer calling it, not communicable, stated, "the immunity of wounded and others mixed with the cholera patients in the hospitals; the immunity of medical men, of attendants, of inspectors, and of the families of the different *employés* attached to the service of cholera patients; the example of a porter, who died of the disease, without his wife or children, who slept in the same bed with him, having been attacked; the example of three women attacked (two of whom died, and one recovered), and the children at their breasts, one of six months, and the other two of twelve, not contracting the disease."

At a subsequent meeting of the Academy, a letter from Dr. Gaymard, one of the Commission to St. Petersburg, was read, in which it was stated, while referring to the comparative mortality at different points there, that, "The cause of this enormous difference was, that the authorities wished to isolate the sick—[Observe this well reader]—and even send them out of the city; now the hospital is on a steep mountain, and, to get to it, the carriages were obliged to take a long circuit through a sandy road, which occupied an hour at least; and if we add to the exposure to the air, the fatigue of this removal, and the time which elapsed after the invasion of the disease, the deplorable state of the patient on his arrival, and the great mortality may be accounted for."

"The progress of the disease was the same as in other places; it was at the moment when it arrived at its height, and when, consequently, the greatest intercourse [Observe reader!] took place with the sick, that the number of attacks wonderfully diminished all at once (*tout à coup*), and without any appreciable cause. The points of the city most distant from each other were invaded. Numbers of families crowded [*entassés*] who had given aid to cholera patients, remained free from the disease, while persons isolated in high and healthy situations [*usually* healthy meant of course] were attacked. It especially attacked the poorer classes, and those given to spirituous liquors. Scarcely twenty persons in easy circumstances were attacked, and even the greater part of these had deviated from a regular system."

The inferences drawn, according to a medical journal, from the whole of Dr. Gaymard's communication, are—

"1. That the system of sanatory measures, adopted in Russia, did not any where stop the disease.

"2. That without entering on the question as to the advantages to be derived from a moral influence arising out of sanatory cordons, placed round a vast state like France, these measures are to be regarded as useless in the interior, in towns, and round houses.

"3. That nothing has been able to obstruct the progressive advance of the disease in a direction from India westward.

"4. That the formation of temporary hospitals, and domiciliary succour, are the only measures which can alleviate this great scourge."

A letter from Dr. Gaymard to Dr. Keraudren was read at the meeting of the Academy, in which it was stated, that in an Hospital at Moscow, in which Dr. Delauny was employed from the month of December, 1830, to the end of December, 1831, 587 cholera patients, and 860 cases of other diseases, were treated—"Not one of the latter was attacked with cholera, although the hospital consists of one building, the coridors communicating with each other, and the same linen serving indiscriminately for all. The attendants did not prove to be more liable to attacks. The relatives were suffered to visit their friends in hospital, and this step produced the best impression on the populace, who remained calm. They can establish at Moscow, that there was not the smallest analogy between the cholera and the plague which ravaged that city in the reign of Catharine." Dr. Gaymard declares, that, having gone to Russia without preconceived ideas on the subject, "he is convinced that interior quarrantines, and the isolation of houses and of sick in towns, has been accompanied by disastrous consequences." Is there yet enough of evidence to shew that this disease is positively *not to be made* communicable from the sick?

Honour still be to those of the profession who, from conscientious and honorable motives, have changed from non-contagionists to contagionists in regard to this disease; and all that should be demanded is, that their *opinions* may not for one moment be suffered to outweigh, on an occasion of vital importance, the great mass of evidence now on record quite in accordance with that just stated. One gentleman of unquestionable respectability gives as a reason (seemingly his very strongest) for a change of opinion, that he has been credibly informed that when the cholera broke out on one side of the street in a certain village in Russia, a medical man had a barrier put up by which the communication with the other side was cut off, and the disease thus, happily, prevented from extending. Now, admitting to the full extent the appearance of the disease on one side of the village only—a thing by the way hitherto as little proved as many others on the contagion side of the question—still, if there be any one thing more striking than another, in the history of the progress of cholera, it is this very circumstance of opposite rows of houses, or of barracks, or bazaars, or lines of camp, being free, while the disease raged in the others, and without any sort of barricading or restriction of intercourse. If people choose to take the trouble to look for the evidence, *plenty* of such is recorded. Now just consider for one moment how this famous Russian story stands: had the barricading begun early, the matter would have stood an examination a little better; but this man of good intentions never thought of his barriers till the one-sided progress of the disease had been manifest enough, *without them:*—and then consider how the communication had existed between both rows before those barriers were put up, and how impossible it was, unless by a file of soldiers, to have debarred all communication:—let all this be considered, and probably the case will stand at its true value, which is, if I may take the liberty of saying so,—just nothing at all. Let us bear in mind the circumstance already quoted from the East India records,—of one company of the 14th Regiment, at the extreme end of a barrack, escaping the disease, almost wholly, while it raged in the other nine; and this without a barrier too. But such circumstances are by no means of rare occurrence in other diseases arising from deteriorated atmosphere. Mr. Wilson, a naval surgeon, has shewn how yellow fever has prevailed *on one side* of a ship, and I have had pointed out to me, by a person who lived near it for thirty years, a spot on this our earth where *ague* attacks only those inhabiting the houses in one particular line, and without any difference as to elevation or other appreciable cause, except that the sun's rays do not impinge equally on both ranges in the morning and evening.

The advancement of the cause of truth has, no doubt, suffered some check in this country, by the announcement that another gentleman of great respectability (Mr. Orton) finds his belief as to non-contagion in cholera a good deal shaken: but we find that this change has not arisen from further personal knowledge of the disease, and if it be from any representations regarding occurrences in Europe, connected with cholera, we have seen how, from almost all quarters, the evidence lies quite on the side of his first opinions. Whatever the change may be owing to, we should continue, as in other cases, not to give an undue preference even to opinions coming from him, to well authenticated facts—facts, among which some particularly strong are still furnished *by himself*, even in the second edition of his book:—"It must be admitted that, in a vast number of instances in India, those persons [medical men and attendants] have suffered no more from the complaint than if they had been attending so many wounded men. This is a fact which, however embarrassing to the medical inquirer, [for our part we cannot see the *embarrassment*] is highly consolatory in a practical point of view, both to him and to all whose close intercourse with the sick is imperatively required."—(*p. 316*)—"We are therefore forced to the conclusion, however, at variance with the common laws of contagion, that in this disease,—at least in India, the most intimate intercourse with the sick is not, in general, productive of more infection than the average quantity throughout the community." (*p. 326*). Let us contrast the statements in the following paragraphs:—"For in all its long and various courses, it may be traced from place to place, and has never, as far as our information extends, started up at distant periods of time and space, leaving any considerable intervening tracts of country untouched." (p. 329)—"All attempts to trace the epidemic to its origin at a point, appears to have failed, and to have shewn that it had not one, but various local sources in the level and alluvial, the marshy and jungly tract of country which forms the delta of the Ganges, and extends from thence to the Burraumposter." (p. 329) Now let us observe what follows regarding the particular *regularity* in the progress of the disease, as just mentioned:—"Another instance of irregularity in its course, even in those provinces where it appears to have been most regular, is stated [now pray observe] in its having skipped from Verdoopatly to a village near Palamacotta, leaving a distance of sixty miles at first unaffected." (p. 332)!!—This is not the way to obtain proselytes I presume.

The situation of our medical brethren at Sunderland is most perplexing, and demands the kindest consideration on the part of the country at large; but let nothing which has occurred disturb the harmony so essential to the general welfare of that place, should their combined efforts be hereafter required on any occasion of public calamity. In truth both parties may be said to be right—the one in stating that the disease in question *is Indian cholera*, because the symptoms are precisely similar—the other that it *is not Indian cholera*, because it exists in Sunderland, and without having been imported—IN NEITHER COUNTRY IS IT COMMUNICABLE FROM ONE PERSON TO ANOTHER, as is now plainly shown upon evidence of a nature which will bear any investigation; and if blame, on account of injury to commerce, be fairly attributable to any, it is to those who, all the world over, pronounced this disease, on grounds the most untenable, a disease of a contagious or communicable nature. Let the Sunderland Board of Health not imagine that their situation is new, for similar odium has fallen *on the first* who told the plain truth, in other instances—at Tortosa, a few years ago, the first physician who announced the appearance of the yellow fever, was, according to different writers, *stoned to death*; and at Barcelona, in 1821, a similar fate had well nigh occurred to Dr. Bahi, one of the most eminent men there—we need not, I presume, fear that a scene of this kind will take place in this country,—though the cries of "no cholera!" and "down with Ogden!" have been heard.

One word as to observations regarding the needlessness of discussing the contagion question: the truth is, that the cleanliness and comfort of the people excepted, you can no more make *other arrangements* with propriety, till this point be settled, than a General can near the enemy by whom he is threatened, till it be ascertained whether that enemy be cavalry or infantry.

My object in these letters is not to obtrude opinions upon the public, being well aware that they cannot be so well entitled as those of many others, to attention; but I wish to place before the public, for their consideration, a collection of facts which I think are likely to be of no small importance at a moment like the present. In addition to the many authorities referred to in the foregoing pages, I would beg to call the public attention to a paper in the *Windsor Express* of the 12th November, by Dr. Fergusson, Inspector General of Hospitals, a gentleman of great experience, and who has given the *coup de grace* to the opinion of contagion in cholera. Indeed the opinion now seems to be virtually abandoned; for, as to quarantine on our ships from Sunderland, it is, perhaps, a thing that cannot be avoided, if the main consideration be *the expediency of the case*, until an arrangement between leading nations takes place. We have seen, in regard to Austria, how the matter stands, and our ships from every port in the country would be refused admission into foreign ports, if we did not subject those from Sunderland to quarantine; which state of things, it is hoped, will now be soon put an end to.

FINIS.

LETTERS

ON THE

CHOLERA MORBUS,

&c. &c. &c.

WINDSOR, FEB. 9, 1832.

Salus populi suprema Lex.

In writing the following letters, which I have given in the order of their respective dates, I was actuated by the state of the public mind at the time in regard to the dreaded disease of which they principally treat. The two first were addressed to the Editor of the WINDSOR EXPRESS, and the third to a Medical Society here, of which I am a member. The contemplation of the subject has beguiled many hours of sickness and bodily pain, and I now commit the result to the press in a more connected form, from the same motives, I believe, that influence other writers—zeal in the cause of truth, whatever that may turn out to be, and predilection for what has flowed from my own pen, not however without the desire and belief, that what I have thus written may prove useful in the discussion of a question which has in no small degree agitated our three kingdoms, and most deeply interested every civilized nation on the face of the earth.

No one, unless he can take it upon him to define the true nature of this new malignant Cholera Morbus, can be warranted utterly to deny the existence of contagion, but he may at the least be permitted to say, that if contagion do exist at all, it must be the weakest in its powers of diffusion, and the safest to approach of any that has ever yet been known amongst diseases. Amateur physicians from the Continent, and from every part of the United Kingdoms, eager and keen for Cholera, and more numerous than the patients themselves, beset and surrounded the sick in Sunderland with all the fearless self-exposing zeal of the missionary character, yet no one could contrive, even in the foulest dens of that sea-port, to produce the disease in his own person, or to carry it in his saturated clothing to the healthier quarters of the town where he himself had his lodging.[17] Surely if the disease had been typhus fever, or any other capable of contaminating the atmosphere of a sick apartment, or giving out infection more directly from the body of a patient, the result must have been different; its course, notwithstanding, has been most unaccountably and peculiarly its own— slow and sure for the most part, the infected wave has rolled on from its tropical origin in the far distant east, to the borders of the arctic circle in the west—not unfrequently in the face of the strongest winds, as if the blighting action of those atmospherical currents had prepared the surface of the earth, as well as the human body for the reception and deposition of the poison; but so far from always following the stream and line of population as has been attempted to be shown, it has often run directly counter to both, seldom or never desolating the large cities of Europe, like the plague and other true contagions, but rather wasting its fury upon encampments of troops, as in the east, or the villages and hamlets of thickly peopled rural districts.

[17] The numbers were so great (to which I should probably have added one had my health permitted) as actually to make gala day in Sunderland, and to call forth a public expression of regret at their departure.

That it could have been descried on no other than the above line must be self-evident, but to say that it has followed it in the manner that a contagious disease ought to have done, in our own country for instance, is at variance with the fact. From Sunderland and Newcastle to the south, the ways were open, the stream of population dense and continuous, the conveyances innumerable, the communications uninterrupted and constant. Towards the thinly-peopled north how different the aspect,—townships rare, the country often high, cold, and dreary, in many parts of the line without inhabitants or the dwellings of man for many miles together, yet does the disease suddenly alight at Haddington, a hundred miles off, without having touched the towns of Berwick, Dunbar, or any of the intermediate places. It is said to have been carried there by vagrant paupers from Sunderland. Can this be true? Could any such with the disease upon them in any shape, have encountered such a winter journey without leaving traces of it in their course?[18] or, if they carried it in their clothing, the winds of the hills must have disinfected these *fomites* long before their arrival. No contagionist, however unscrupulous and enthusiastic, nor quarantine authority however vigilant, can pretend to say how the disease has been introduced at the different points of Sunderland, Haddington, and Kirkintulloch,—no more than he can tell why it has appeared at Doncaster, Portsmouth, and an infinity of other places without spreading. Even now, it lingers at the gates of the great open cities of Edinburgh and Glasgow, as if like a malarious disease, (which I by no means say that it is) it better found its food in the hamlet and the tent, in fact, amongst the inhabitants of ground tenements, than in paved towns and stone buildings. We must go farther and acknowledge, that for many months past our atmosphere has been tainted with the miasm or poison of Cholera Morbus, as manifested by unusual cases of the disease almost everywhere, and that these harbingers of the pestilence only wanted such an ally as the drunken jubilee at Gateshead, or atmospherical conditions and changes of which we know nothing, to give it current and power. That the epidemic current of disease wherever men exist and congregate together, must, in the first instance, resemble the contagious so strongly as to make it impossible to distinguish the one from the other, must be self-evident; and it is only after the touchstone has been applied, and proof of non-communicability been obtained, as at Sunderland, that the impartial observer can be enabled to discern the difference.—Still, however, must he be puzzled with the inexplicable phenomena of this strange pestilence, but if he feel himself at a loss for an argument against contagion, he has only to turn to one of the most recent communications from the Central Board of Health, where he will find that "That the subsidiary force under Col. Adams, which arrived in perfect health *in the neighbourhood* of a village of India infected with Cholera, had seventy cases of the disease the night of its arrival, and twenty deaths the next day," as if the march under a tropical sun, and the encampment upon malarious ground, or beneath a poisoned atmosphere, were all to go for nothing; and that the neighbourhood of an infected village, with which it is not stated that they held communication, had in that instantaneous manner alone, produced the disease. This is surely drawing too largely upon our credulity, and practising upon our fears beyond the mark.

[18] The Cholera in this country would appear always to travel with the pedestrian, and to eschew the stage coach even as an outside passenger.

The anti-contagionist, in acknowledging his ignorance, leaves the question open to examination; but the contagionist has solved the problem to his own mind, and closed the field of investigation, without, however, ceasing to denounce the antagonist who would disturb a conclusion which has given him so much contentment.—Let us here examine, for a moment, who in this case best befriends his fellow men. The latter, in vindication of a principle which he cannot prove, would shut the book of enquiry, sacrifice and abandon the sick, (for to this it must ever come the moment pestilential contagion is proclaimed,) extinguish human sympathy in panic fear, and sever every tie of domestic life,—the other would wait for proofs before he proclaimed the ban, and even then, with pestilence steaming before him, would doubt whether that pestilence could be best extinguished, or whether it would not be aggravated into ten-fold virulence, by excommunicating the sick.

In my first letter I have endeavoured to unveil the mystery and fallacy of fumigations, for which our government has paid so dear,[19] and in place of the chemical disinfectants so much extolled, of the applicability of which we know nothing, and which have always failed whenever they were depended upon, have recommended the simple and sure ones of heat, light, water, and air, with one exception, the elements of our forefathers, which combined always with all possible purity of atmosphere, person, and habitation, have been found as sure and certain in effect as they are practical and easy of application.

[19] Parliament voted a reward of £5000 to Doctor Carmichael Smith for the discovery.

Of our quarantine laws I have spoken freely, because I believe their present application, in many instances, to be unnecessary cruel and mischievous. Too long have they been regarded as an engine of State, connected with vested interests and official patronage, against which it was unsafe to murmur, however pernicious they might be to commerce, or discreditable to a country laying claim to medical knowledge. The regulation for preventing the importation of tropical yellow fever, (which is altogether a malarious disease of the highest temperature of heat and unwholesome locality,) into England or even into Gibraltar, stands eminent for absurdity. It has long been denounced by abler pens than mine, and I know not how it can be farther exposed, unless we could induce the inhabitants of our West India Colonies to enforce the lex talionis, and institute quarantines, which they might do with the same or better reason, against the importation of pleurises and catarrhs from the colder regions of Europe; a practical joke of this kind has been known to succeed after reason, argument, and evidence, amounting to the most palpable demonstration, had proved of no avail.

While I have thus impugned the authority of boards and missions, and establishments, I trust it never can be imputed to me that I could have intended any, the smallest personal allusion, to the eminent and estimable men of whom they are composed,—all such I utterly disclaim; and to the individual, in particular, who presided over our mission to Russia, who has been my colleague in the public service, and whose friendship I have enjoyed from early youth, during a period of more than forty years, I would here, were it the proper place, pay the tribute of respect which the usefulness of his life, and excellence of his character, deserves.

LETTER I.
TO THE EDITOR OF THE WINDSOR EXPRESS.

Sir,—Being well aware of the handsome manner in which you have always opened the columns of your liberal journal to correspondents upon every subject of public interest, I make no further apology for addressing through the WINDSOR EXPRESS, some observations to the inhabitants of Windsor and its neighbourhood upon the all-engrossing subject of Cholera Morbus.

That pestilence, despite of quarantine laws, boards of health, and sanatory regulations, has now avowedly reached our shores, and we may be permitted at last to acknowledge the presence of the enemy—to describe to the affrighted people the true nature of the terrors with which he is clothed—and to point out how these can be best combatted or avoided.

That the seeds of his fury have long been sown amongst us may be proved, and will be proved, ere long, by reference to fatal cases of unwonted Cholera Morbus appearing, occasionally during the last six months, in London, Port Glasgow, Abingdon, Hull, and many other places, which, as it did not spread, have been passed unheeded by our health conservators; but, had the poison then been sufficiently matured to give it epidemic current, would have been blazed forth as imported pestilence. Some one or other of the ships constantly arriving from the north of Europe could easily have been fixed upon as acting the part of Pandora's box, and smugglers from her dispatched instanter to carry the disease into the inland quarters of the kingdom. I write in this manner, not from petulance, but from the analogy of the yellow fever, where this very game I am now describing, has so often been played with success in the south of Europe; and will be played off again, for so long as lucrative boards of health and gainful quarantine establishments, with extensive influence and patronage, shall continue to be resorted to for protection against a non-existent—an impossible contagion.

But to the disease in question.—It must have had a spontaneous origin somewhere, and that origin has been clearly traced to a populous unhealthy town in the East Indies—no infection was ever pretended to have been carried there, yet, it devastated with uncontroulable fury, extending from district to district, but in the most irregular and unaccountable manner, sparing the unwholesome localities in its immediate neighbourhood, yet attacking the more salubrious at a distance—passing by the most populous towns in its direct course at one time, but returning to them in fury at another, staying in none, however crowded, yet attacking all some time or other, until almost every part of the Indian peninsula had experienced its visitation.

There is an old term, as old as the good old English physician, Sydenham— *constitution of the atmosphere*—and to what else than to some inscrutable condition of the element in which we live, and breathe, and have our being—in fact to an atmospheric poison beyond our ken, can we ascribe the terrific gambols of such a destroyer. 'Tis on record, that when our armies were serving in the pestilential districts of India, hundreds, without any noticeable warning, would be taken ill in the course of a single night, and thousands in the course of a few days, in one wing of the army, while the other wing, upon different ground, and consequently under a different current of atmosphere, although in the course of the regular necessary communication between troops in the field, would remain perfectly free from the disease. It would then cease as suddenly and unaccountably as it began,—attacking, weeks after, the previously unscathed division of the army, or not attacking it at all at the time, yet returning at a distant interval, when all traces of the former epidemic had ceased, and committing the same devastation. Now, will any man, not utterly blinded by prejudice, candidly reviewing these facts, pretend to say, that this could be a personal contagion, cognizable by, and amenable to, any of the known or even supposable laws of infection—that the hundreds of the night infected one another, or that the thousands of the few days owed their disease to personal communication,—as well affect to believe that the African Simoon, which prostrates the caravan, and leaves the bones of the traveller to whiten in the sandy desert, could be a visitation of imported pestilence.

It may then be asked, have we no protection against this fearful plague? No means of warding it off? Certainly none against its visitation! It will come— it will go; we can neither keep it out, or retain it, if we wished, amongst us. The region of its influence is above us and beyond our controul; and we might as well pretend to arrest the influx of the swallows in summer, and the woodcocks in the winter season, by cordons of troops and quarantine regulations, as by such means to stay the influence, of an atmospheric poison; but in our moral courage, in our improved civilization, in the perfecting of our medical and health police, in the generous charitable spirit of the higher orders, assisting the poorer classes of the community, in the better condition of those classes themselves, compared with the poor of other countries, and in the devoted courage and assistance of the medical profession every where, we shall have the best resources. Trusting to these, it has been found that, in countries far less favoured than ours, wherever the impending pestilence has only threatened a visitation, there the panic has been terrible, and people have even died of fear; but when it actually arrived, and they were obliged to look it in the face, they found, that by putting their trust in what I have just laid down, they were in comparative safety; that, the destitute, the uncleanly, above all, the intemperate and the debauched,   were   almost its only victims; that the epidemic poison, whatever it might be, had strength to prevail only against those who had been previously unnerved by fear, or weakened by debauchery; and that moral courage, generous but temperate living, and regularity of habits in every respect, proved nearly a certain safe-guard. They found further, that quarantine regulations were worse than useless—that the gigantic military organization of Russia—the rigorous military despotism of Prussia—and the all-searching police of Austria, with their walled towns, and guards and gates, and cordons of troops, were powerless against this unseen pestilence, and that as soon as the quarantine laws were relaxed, and free communication allowed, the disease assumed a milder character, and speedily disappeared.

I say, then, confidently, that Cholera Morbus never will commit ravages in this country, beyond the bounds of the worst purlieus of society, unless it be fostered into infectious, pestilential activity, by the absurd, however well-meant, measures of the conservative boards of health, such as have been just recommended in what has always been esteemed the most influential, best-informed journal of England, I mean the QUARTERLY REVIEW. If the writer of the article who recommends the enforcement of the ancient quarantine laws in all their strictness, be a medical man, he surely ought to know, that wherever human beings are confined and congregated together in undue numbers, more especially if they be in a state of disease, there the matter of contagion, the typhoid principle, the septic (putrefactive) human poison or by what other name it may be called, is infallibly generated and extends itself, but in its own impure atmosphere only, as a personal infection to those who approach it, under the form and features of the prevailing epidemic, whatever that may be. Hence we have all heard of contagious pleurisies, catarrhs, dysenteries, ulcers, &c., and if the doctrines of that writer be received, we shall soon also hear of contagious Cholera Morbus with a vengeance. His exhortations would go to shut up the sick from human intercourse, to proclaim the ban of society against them, and under the most pitiable circumstances of bodily distress, to proscribe them as objects of terror and danger, instead of being as they actually are, helpless innocuous fellow creatures, calling loudly for our promptest succour and commiseration in their utmost need. They would go further to array man against his fellow man in all the cruel selfishness of panic terror, sever the dearest domestic ties, paralize commerce, suspend manufactures, and destroy the subsistance of thousands, and all for the gratification of a prejudice which has been proved to be utterly baseless in every country of Europe from Archangel to Hamburgh and Sunderland. Happily for our country, these measures are now as absurd and impracticable as they would be tyrannical and unjust. They could not be borne even under the despotic military sway of Prussia and Russia, and in this free country it would be impossible to enforce them for a single week. The very attempt would at once, throughout the whole land, produce confusion and misery incalculable.

I say, on the contrary, throw open their dwellings to the free air of heaven, the best cordial and diluent of foul atmosphere in every disease—let their fellow townsmen hasten to carry them food, fuel, cordials, cloathing, and bedding, speak to them the words of consolation, and should they have fear to approach the sick, I take it upon me to say, they will be accompanied by any and every medical practitioner of the place, who, in their presence, will minister to the afflicted, inspire their breath, and perform every other professional office of humanity, without the smallest fear or risk of infection; for they read the daily records of their profession, where it has been proved to them, that in the open but crowded hospitals of Warsaw, under the most embarrassing circumstances of warfare and disease, out of a hundred medical men, with their assistants and attendants, frequenting the sick wards of Cholera, not one took the disease; that, for the sake of proving its nature, they even went so far as to clothe themselves with the vestments of the dying, to sleep in the beds of the recently dead, and to innoculate themselves in every way with the blood and fluids of the worst cases, without, in a single instance, producing Cholera Morbus.[20] The accounts may not, indeed, cannot be the same from every other quarter, for medical men must be as liable to fall under the influence of an atmospherical epidemic disease as other classes of the community; but the above fact is alone sufficient to prove that it cannot be a personal contagion.

[20] Vide Medical Gazette.

Even should that worst of true contagions, the plague of the Levant, which every nation is bound to guard against, despite of all our precautions, be introduced amongst us, measures better calculated for the destruction of a community, could scarcely be devised, than the ancient quarantine regulations; for they certainly would convert every house proscribed by their mark, into a den and focus of the most concentrated pestilential contagion, ensuring fearful retribution upon those who had thus so blindly shut them up. The mark alone, besides being equivalent to a sentence of death upon all the inmates, would effect all this—the sick would be left to die unassisted, unpurified, uncleansed amidst their accumulated contagion, and the dead, as has happened before, lie unburied or scarcely covered in, till they putrified in pestiferous heaps. Most certainly it would be proper and beneficial, even a duty, for all who could afford the means, and were not detained by public duties, to fly the place, and equally proper for the other residents who continued in health, to segregate themselves as they best could.—Plenty of free labour amongst those who must ever work for their daily bread, would still remain for all municipal purposes, and these our rulers, so far from consenting thus to proscribe the sick, should employ openly in giving them every succour and aid, under the direction and with instructions of safety from a well arranged medical police. It would not be difficult to show, that the mortality, during the last great plague in London, was increased a hundred fold, by following the very measures now recommended in these regulations; and, that the barbarous predestinarian Turk, in the very head quarters of the plague itself, who despises all regulation, but attends his sick friend to the last, never yet brought down upon his country such calamitous visitations of pestilence, as enlightened Christian nations have inflicted upon themselves, by ill-judged laws. The Turk, to be sure, by rejecting all precaution, and admitting, without scruple, infection into his ports, sees Constantinople invaded by the plague every year; but, when not preposterously interfered with, it passes away, even amongst that wretched population, like a common epidemic, without leaving any remarkable traces of devastation behind it: and surely to establish and make a pest-house of the dwelling of every patient who might be discovered or even suspected to be ill, would be most preposterous. The writing on the wall would not be more apalling to the people, and scarcely less fatal to the object, than the cry of mad dog in the streets, with this difference, that when the dog was killed, the scene would be closed, but the proscribed patient would remain, even in his death and after it, to avenge the wrong.

But sufficient to the day is the evil thereof, the question is now of Cholera Morbus; I am willing to meet any objection, and the most obvious one that can be offered to me, (if it be not an imported disease) is its first appearance in our commercial sea-ports. To this I might answer, that it has been hovering over us, making occasional stoops, for the last six months, even in the most inland parts of the country; but I will waive that advantage, and meet it on plainer grounds of argument and truth.—An atmospherical poison must evidently possess the greatest influence, where it finds the human race under the most unfavourable circumstances of living, habits, locality, and condition. Now, where can these be met with so obviously as in our large sea-port towns on the lowest levels of the country, and in their crowded alleys, always near to the harbour for the shipping? There the disease, if its seeds existed in the atmosphere, would be most likely to break out in preference to all other situations; and if at the time of its so appearing, ships should arrive, as they are constantly doing from all parts of the world, whose crews, according to the custom of sailors, plunge instantly into drunkenness and debauchery, and present as it were, ready prepared, the very subjects the pestilence was waiting for; how easy then, for an alarmed or prejudiced board of health to point out the supposed importing vessel, and freight her with a cargo of the new pestilence from any part of the world they may choose to fix upon. This is no imaginary case; it was for long of annual occurrence with respect to the yellow fever, both in the West Indies and North America. "There our thoughtless intemperate sailors were not only the first to suffer from the epidemic, in its course or about to begin, but they were denounced as the importers, by the prejudiced vulgar, and the accusation was loudly re-echoed even amongst the better informed, by all who wished to make themselves believe that pestilence could not be a native product of their own atmosphere and habitations."Before I have done, I feel called upon to say a few words upon the efficacy of fumigation as a preservative against Cholera Morbus and other infectious diseases. In regard to the first the question is settled. In Russia, throughout Germany, and I believe everywhere else in Europe, they were productive of no good, they did mischief, and were therefore discontinued. This has been verified by reports from the seats of the disease everywhere. In regard to other contagions I can speak, not without knowledge, at least not without experience, for it was the business and the duty of my military life, during a long course of years, to see them practised in ships, barracks, hospitals, and cantonements, and I can truly declare I never saw contagion in the smallest degree arrested by them, and that disease never failed to spread, and follow its course unobstructed, and unimpeded by their use. In the well-conditioned houses of the affluent where ventilation and cleanliness are matters of habit and domestic discipline, they may be a harmless plaything during the prevalence of scarlet fever and such like infections, or even do a little good by inspiring the attendants with confidence, however false, as a preservative against contagion; but in the confined dwellings of the poor they are positively mischievous, because they cannot be used without shutting out the wholesome atmospheric air, and substituting for it a factitious gas, which for aught we know, or can know of the nature of the contagious vapour, whether acid, alkaline, or anything else, may actually be adding to its deleterious principle instead of neutralising it: but in thus striking away a prop from the confidence of the poor, I thank God I can furnish them with other preservatives and disinfectants, which I take it upon me to say, they will find as simple and practicable as they are infallible. For the first, the liberal use of cold water and observance of free ventilation, with slaked lime to wash the walls, and quick lime when they can get it, to purify their dung heaps and necessaries, are among the best; but when actually infected, then heat is the only purificator yet known of an infected dwelling. Let boiling water be plentifully used to every part of the house and article of furniture to which it can be made applicable. Let portable iron stoves, filled with ignited charcoal only, be placed in the apartment closely shut, and the heat kept up for a few hours to any safe degree of not less than 120° Farenheit, and let foul infected beds and mattresses be placed in a baker's oven heated to the same,[21] and my life for it no infection can after that possibly adhere to houses, clothes, or furniture. The living fountain of infection from the patient himself, constantly giving out the fresh material, cannot of course be so closed, but whether he lives or dies, if the above be observed, he will leave no infection behind him.[22]

[21] The oven on that account need not lose character with bread-eaters, for according to the old adage, Omne vitium per ignem excoquitur.

[22] Light too, more especially when assisted by a current of atmospheric air, is a true and sure disinfectant, but it is not so applicable as heat in the common contagions, from requiring an exposure of the infected substances for days together, or even a longer period, before it can be made effective.

It is now time to bring this tedious letter to a close; I shall be happy, through the same channel, to give any information, or answer any inquiries that may be authenticated by the signature of the writer; but anonymous writing of any kind, I shall not consider myself bound to notice. Should the dreaded disease spread its ravages throughout our population, I may then, at some future early opportunity, trusting to your indulgence, trespass again upon your columns with further communications on this most interesting subject.

WILLIAM FERGUSSON,
Inspector-General of Hospitals.

P.S.—Throughout the foregoing letter, I have used the words contagion and infection as precisely synonymous terms, meaning communicability of disease from one person to another.

November 9, 1831.

LETTER II.
TO THE EDITOR OF THE WINDSOR EXPRESS.

Sir,—In my last letter, I treated of the practicability of guarding our country against the now European and Continental disease, malignant Cholera Morbus, by quarantine regulations. In the present one, it is my intention still in a popular manner to scrutinise more deeply, the doctrine of imported contagions; to point out, if I can, those true contagions which can be warded off by our own exertions, in contradistinction to others which are altogether beyond our controul; and here it may be as well to premise, that when I use the term epidemic, I mean atmospheric influence, endemic-terrestrial influence, or emanation from the soil; and by pestilential, I mean the spread of malignant disease without any reference to its source. The terms contagion and infection have already been explained.

It must be evident, that legislative precaution can only be made applicable to the first of these. The last being unchangeable by human authority, are not to be assailed by any decrees we can fulminate against them; and if it can be shown, which it has been by our best and latest reports, that Cholera Morbus eminently and indisputably belongs to that class—that the strictest cordons of armed men could not avail to save the towns of the continent, nor the strictest quarantine our own shores, from its invasion—it surely must be time to cease those vain attempts, to lay down the arms that have proved so useless, and turn our undivided attention, now that it has fairly got amongst us, to conservative police, and the treatment of the disease; but as the contagionists still insist that it was imported from Hamburgh to Sunderland, it behoves us to clear away this preliminary difficulty before proceeding to other points of the enquiry.

I take it for granted, that ships proceeding from Sunderland to Hamburgh could only be colliers, and that according to the custom of such vessels, they returned, as they do from the port of London, light; and I admit, that on or about the time of their return, Cholera Morbus, under the severe form which characterises the Asiatic disease, made its appearance in that port, presenting a fair *prima facie* case of imported contagion; but as at the period of its thus breaking out in Sunderland, a case equally as fatal and severe shewed itself, according to the public accounts, in the upper part of Newcastle, 10 miles off; another equally well-marked, in a healthy quarter in Edinburgh; a third, not long before in Rugby, in the very centre of the kingdom; and a fourth in Sunderland itself, as far back as the month of August, as well as many others in different parts of the country;[23] it became incumbent on the quarantine authorities, indeed upon all men interested in the question, whether contagionists or otherwise, to shew the true state of these vessels, as well as of the cases above alluded to, and whether the Cholera Morbus had ever been on board of them, either at Hamburgh or during the homeward voyage, so as by any possibility they could have introduced the disease into an English port. Now will any person pretend to say that this has been done, or that it could not have been done, or deny that it was a measure, which, if properly executed, would have thrown light upon the true character of the disease, not only for the information of our own government but of every government in Europe; that deputations from the Board of Health, backed and supported by all the power and machinery of government, with the suspected ships locked up in quarantine, and the persons of the crews actually in their power, could not have verified to the very letter, the history of every hour and day of their health, from the moment of their arrival at Hamburgh till their return into port? This measure was so obviously and imperiously called for, as constituting the only rational ground on which the importing contagionists could stand, or their opponents meet them in argument, that after having waited in vain for the report, I raised my own feeble voice in the only department to which I had access, urging an immediate, though then late, investigation. No good cause, having truth for its basis, could have been so overlooked, and without unfairness or illiberality, we are irresistibly forced to the conclusion, that had the enquiry (the only one, by the bye, worth pursuing, as bearing directly on the question at issue) been pushed to the proof, it would have shown the utter nullity of quarantine guards against atmospherical pestilence, the thorough baselessness of the doctrine of importation.

[23] Two of a type most unusual for this country, and the Winter Season, have occurred in the vale of the Thames, not far from here, which, as they both recovered, and the disease did not spread in any way, were very properly allowed to pass without sounding any alarm, but the gentleman who attended one of the cases, and had been familiar with the disease in India, at once recognized it again, in its principal distinguishing features.

Without entering into the miserable disputes on this subject, which, amidst a tissue of fable and prejudice, self-interest and misrepresentation, have so often disgraced the medical profession at Gibraltar; I shall now proceed to shew, by reference to general causes, how baseless and mischievous have been the same doctrines and authority when exercised in that part of the British dominions:—

Within the last thirty years, yellow fever has, at least four times, invaded the fortress of Gibraltar; during which time also, the population of its over-crowded town has more than quadrupled, presenting as fair a field, for the generation within, or reception from without, of imported pestilence as can well be imagined,—yet plague, the truest of all contagions, typhus fever, and other infectious diseases, have never prevailed, as far as I know, amongst them. The plague of the Levant has not been there, I believe, for 150 years; yet Gibraltar, the free port of the Mediterranean, open to every flag, stands directly in the course of the only maritime outlet, from its abode and birth-place in the east, being in fact, to use the language of the road, the house of call for the commerce of all nations coming from the upper Mediterranean. Now, can there be a more obvious inference from all this, than that the plague, being a true contagion, may be kept off without difficulty, by ordinary quarantine precautions; but the other being an endemic malarious disease, generated during particular seasons, within the garrison itself, and the offspring of its own soil, is altogether beyond their controul. The malarious or marsh poison, which in our colder latitudes produces common ague, in the warmer, remittent fever, and in unfavourable southern localities of Europe, (such as those of crowded towns, where the heat has been steadily for some time of an intertropical degree)—true yellow fever, which is no more than the highest grade of malarious disease; but this has never occurred in European towns, unless during the driest seasons—seasons actually blighted by drought, when hot withering land winds have destroyed surface vegetation, and as in the locality of Gibraltar, have left the low-lying becalmed, and leeward town to corrupt without perflation or ventilation amidst its own accumulated exhalations. I know not how I can better illustrate the situation of Gibraltar in these pestiferous seasons, than by a quotation from a report of my own on the Island of Guadaloupe, in the year 1816, which, though written without any possible reference to the question at issue, has become more apposite than anything else I could advance; "all regular currents of wind have the effect of dispersing malaria; when this purifying influence is with-held, either through the circumstances of season, or when it cannot be made to sweep the land on account of the intervention of high hills, the consequences are most fatal. The leeward shores of Guadaloupe, for a course of nearly 30 miles, under the shelter of a very steep ridge of volcanic mountains, never felt the sea breeze, nor any breeze but the night land-wind from the mountains; *and though the soil, which I have often examined, is a remarkably open, dry and pure one, being mostly sand and gravel, altogether, and positively without marsh, in the most dangerous places, it is inconceivably pestiferous throughout the whole tract, and in no place more so than the bare sandy beach near the high-water mark.* The coloured people alone ever venture to inhabit it; and when they see strangers tarrying on the shore after nightfall, they never fail to warn them of their danger. The same remark holds good in regard to the greater part of the leeward coasts of Martinique, *and the leeward alluvial bases and recesses*[24] *of hills, in whatever port of the torrid zone they may be placed*, with the exception, probably of the immediate sites of towns, where the pavements prevent the rain-water being absorbed into the soil, and hold it up to speedy evaporation." Now, conceive a populous crowded town placed in this situation, and you have exactly what Gibraltar and the other towns of Spain and North America, liable to yellow fever, must become in such seasons as I have above described, only, that as they grow more populous and crowded, the danger must be greater, and its visitations more frequent, unless the internal health police be made to keep pace in improvement, with the increasing population.

[24] The leeward niches and recesses of hills, however dry and rocky, become in these seasons of drought, absolute dens of malaria, this will be found proven in my reports made especially of the islands of Dominique and Trinidad, which may be seen at the Army Medical Board Office.

Now in the name of injured commerce—of the deluded people of England—of medical science—of truth and humanity—what occasion can their be to institute an expensive quarantine against such a state of things as this, which can only be mitigated by domestic health police; or why conjure up the unreal phantom of an imported plague, to delude the unhappy sufferers, as much in regard to the true nature of the disease, as to the measures best calculated for their own preservation; when it must be evident that the pestilence has sprung from amidst themselves, and that had it been an external contagion in any degree, the ordinary quarantine, as in case of the plague, would certainly have kept it off; but the question of the contagion of yellow fever, so important to commerce and humanity; and which, like the Cholera, has more than once been used to alarm the coasts of England, demands yet further investigation.

For nearly 40 years have the medical departments of our army and navy been furnished with evidence, from beyond the Atlantic, that this disease possessed no contagious property whatever. These proofs now lie recorded by hundreds in their respective offices, and I take it upon me to say, they will not be found contradicted by more than one out of a hundred, amongst all the reports from the West Indies, which is as much the birth-place of the yellow fever, as Egypt is of the plague: yet, in the face of such a mass of evidence, as great or greater probably than ever was accumulated upon any medical question, has our Government been deluded, to vex commerce with unnecessary restraints, to inflict needless cruelties upon commercial communities, (for what cruelty can be greater than after destroying their means of subsistence by quarantine laws, to pen them up in a den of pestilence, there to perish without escape, amidst their own malarious poison?) and to burden the country with the costs of expensive quarantine establishments. Surely if these departments had done their duty, or will now do it, in so far as to furnish our rulers with an abstract of that evidence, with or without their own opinions, for opinions are as dust in the balance when put in competition with recorded facts, it must be impossible that the delusion could be suffered to endure for another year; or should they unluckily fail thereby to produce conviction on Government, they can refer to the records of commerce, and of our transport departments, which will shew, if enquiry be made, that no ship, however deeply infected before she left the port, (and all ships were uniformly so infected wherever the pestilence raged) ever yet produced, or was able to carry a case of yellow fever beyond the boundaries of the tropics, on the homeward voyage, and that therefore the stories of conveying it beyond seas to Gibraltar, must have been absolutely chimerical. It would indeed, have been a work of supererrogation, little called for, for I think I have fully shown that Gibraltar must be abundantly qualified to manufacture yellow fever for herself.

No less chimerical will be the attempt to shut out Cholera Morbus from our shores by quarantine laws, because throughout Europe, ready prepared, alarmed, and in arms against it, they have succeeded nowhere; whereas, had it been a true contagion and nothing else, they must, with ordinary care, have succeeded everywhere; the disease, as if in mockery, broke through the cordons of armed men, sweeping over the walls of fortified towns, and following its course, even across seas, to the shores of Britain; and yet we are still pretending to oppose it with these foiled weapons.

We are indeed told, by authority, that its appearance in towns has always been coincident with the arrival of barges from inland, or by ships from the sea, but if it be not shown at the same time that the crews of these barges had been infected with the disease, or if, as at Sunderland, no person on board the ships can be identified as having introduced it, while we know that the disease actually was there two months before, we may well ask at what time of the year barges and ships do not arrive in a commercial seaport, or where an epidemic disease, during pestiferous seasons could be more likely to break out than where the most likely subjects are thrown into the most likely places for its explosion, such as newly arrived sailors in an unwholesome seaport, where the license of the shore, or the despondency of quarantine imprisonment must equally dispose them to become its victims.—Besides, what kind of quarantine can we possibly establish with the
 smallest chance of being successful against men who have not got, and never had the disease. Merchandise has been declared incapable of conveying the infection,[25] and are we to interdict the hulls and rigging of Vessels bearing healthy crews, or are we to shut our ports at once against all commerce with the North of Europe, and would this prove successful if we did? a reference to a familiar epidemic will I think at once answer this question.

[25] Vide Russian Ukase.

It is only three months ago that the epidemic Catarrh or Influenza spread throughout the land, travelling like the Cholera in India, when it went up the monsoon, without regard to the East wind; and what could be more likely than the blighting drying process of such a wind, in either the one or the other case, to prepare the body for falling under the influence of whatever disease might be afloat in the atmosphere. In general this passing disease can be distinctly traced, as having affected our continental neighbours on the other side of the channel before ourselves: now can it be supposed that any quarantine could have prevented its first invasion, or arrested its farther progress amongst us. How ridiculous would have been the attempt, and yet with the experience of all Europe before us, have we been enacting that very part with the Cholera Morbus: but further, the same authority which calls for the establishment of quarantine in our ports, tells us that neither proximity nor contact with the sick,[26] is requisite for the production of the disease: now can anything further be wanting beyond this admission, to prove that it must be an epidemic atmospherical poison, and not a personal contagion, and that, under such circumstances, the establishment of quarantine against persons and goods, would manifestly be absurd and uncalled for. So fully satisfied has the Austrian Government been made by experience, of the futility and cruelty of such quarantines, that the Emperor apologises to his subjects for having inflicted them. The King of Prussia makes a similar *amende*, and the Emperor of Russia convinced by the same experience, abolished or greatly relaxed his quarantines several mouths ago.

[26] Vide Reports from Russia.

I am by no means prepared to assert, because I cannot possibly know to the contrary, although from the analogy of other disease I do not believe it, that the Cholera Morbus may not become contagious under certain conditions of the atmosphere, but these cannot be made subject to quarantine laws, and I am fully prepared to acknowledge, that as in the case of other epidemics, it may be made contagious through defective police; but independent of these, it possesses other powers and qualities of self-diffusion, which we can neither understand nor controul. Such, however, is not the case with that other phantom of our quarantine laws—the yellow fever—which can never, under any circumstances of atmosphere, without the aid of the last be made a contagious disease. I speak thus decisively from my experience of its character, as one of the survivors of the St. Domingo war, where, in a period of little more than four years, nearly 700 British commissioned officers, and 30,000 men were swept away by its virulence; as also from subsequent experience, after an interval of 20 years, when in the course of time and service, I became principal medical officer of the windward and leeward colonies, and in that capacity, surveyed and reported upon the whole of these transatlantic possessions.

It was my intention, in these times of panic, to designate to my countrymen, in as far as I could, the true essential intrinsic contagions of the British Isles, (for such there are, and terrible ones too,) which prevail under all circumstances of season, atmosphere, and locality, as contradistinguished from the factitious ones, of our own creating, and the imaginary or false which often spread epidemically, (for there may be an epidemic as well as contagious current of disease)[27] although they possess no contagious property whatever; as well as the foreign contagions, which if we relax in due precaution, may, at any time, be introduced amongst us— but the unreasonable length of this letter, for a newspaper communication, warns me to stop.

[27] For as long as men congregate together, and every supposable degree of communication must of necessity be constantly taking place amongst them, to distinguish a spreading epidemic from a contagious disease when it first breaks out, must obviously be a matter of impossibility; and upon this point the contagionists and their antagonists may rail for ever,—the one will see nothing but contagion, whether in the dead or the living body, and the other will refer every fresh case to atmospheric or terrestrial influence, and both with as much apparent reason as they possibly could desire: but the candid impartial investigator, who waits to observe the course of the disease before coming to a conclusion, and refers to the facts furnished in the Cholera Hospitals of Warsaw and the sick quarters of Sunderland, will never be deceived in regard to its real nature, nor propagate the appalling belief that Cholera Morbus can be made a transportable and transmissible contagion.

I have written thus earnestly, because I deeply feel what I have here put down. It is possible I may have made mistakes, but if I have, they are not intentional, and I shall be happy to be corrected, for I do not live at the head quarters of communication, and my broken health prevents my frequenting in person, the field of investigation. In candour I ought to declare, that the establishment of quarantine against this new and hideous pestilence in the first instance, was the most sacred duty of Government, but now that its true character has been made known, and the futility of quarantine restrictions demonstrated, I feel equally bound, as one of the lieges, to enter my humble protest against their continuance.

Should I write again, I shall still adopt the same popular style, for no other can be adapted to a newspaper communication, and the subject-matter is as interesting to the public, and every head of a family, as it can be to the professional reader; and, in thus making use of your columns, as I can have no motive but that of ardent research after truth, I know that I may always rely upon your assistance and co-operation.

WILLIAM FERGUSSON,
Inspector-General of Hospitals.

Windsor, Nov. 26, 1831.

LETTER III.
TO THE MEDICAL SOCIETY OF WINDSOR.

In this paper it is my intention to treat of the contagious diseases of the British Isles, as well as to offer to the Society some observations on malignant Cholera Morbus, and the mode of its propagation from the tropical regions, where it first arose, to the colder latitudes of Europe.

Having already published two letters on this last part of my subject, I need not here take up your time in recapitulating their contents, but proceed to the consideration of some remaining points of the enquiry; which I find I have either overlooked, or not been so explicit in illustration, as I otherwise might, had I been addressing a body of professional men, instead of the community where I live, with the view of *disabusing* their minds from the effects of irrational panic, and opening their eyes to what I deemed true measures of preservation against the impending disease; and here I may as well add that when I wrote in a newspaper and adopted the style suited to such a channel of communication, I knew none so likely to attract the attention of those influential men, who might possess the power and the will, when disabused of prejudice, to enforce proper laws, instead of running the course that had already been imposed upon them, by men interested in the upholding of our quarantine establishments, or by prejudiced, however well meaning, Boards of Health.

In looking over those letters, I find that the points most open to dispute are the course of the disease throughout the Indian peninsula, and its progress to the frontiers of Russia; as well as its supposed infectious nature, and mode of propagation by human intercourse. In regard to the first, there is no contagionist however avowed and uncompromising, who does not admit that this erratic disease did not often wander from its straight line when the most promising fields lay directly before it; or stop short most unaccountably in its progress, when the richest harvest of victims seemed actually within its jaws—that its course was circuitous when, according to the laws of contagion, it ought to have been straight,—that it refused its prey at one time, and returned to it at another, in a manner that showed its progress was governed by laws which we could neither understand nor controul; and if we search the reports of contagionist writers, we shall find fully as much, and as strong evidence of its progress being independent of human intercourse, as of its being propagated and governed by the laws of contagion.[28]

[28] Vide Orton, Kennedy, &c.

To the question, which has so often been triumphantly asked, of its progress to the Russian frontiers being conducted by caravans along the great highways of human intercourse, and what else than contagion could cause it to be so carried? An admirable journalist has already replied by asking in his turn, on what other line than amongst the haunts of men could we possibly have found, or detected a human disease? And surely the question is most pertinent, for in those barbarous regions that interpose between Russia and India, where the wolf and the robber hold divided alternate sway, and isolated man dares not fix his habitation, but must congregate for safety; where else than in those great thoroughfares could the disease have found its food; or if beyond these, man, almost as ignorant and as savage as the wolf, could have been found; who under such circumstances would have recognised, described, and testified to its existence? Even at Sunderland, amongst ourselves, its existence was long hotly disputed by the learned of the faculty; and the fatalist barbarian of these regions would have dismissed the enquiry with a prayer of resignation, while he bowed his head to the grave, or if his strength permitted, with a stroke of his dagger against the impious enquirer who had dared to interfere with the immutable decrees of fate. The stories too of its importation into Russia, are exactly the same as have come to us from our own Gibraltar, in the case of the yellow fever, and may be expected to come from every other quarter where a well paid officious quarantine is established to find infection in its own defence, and to trace its course in proof of their own services and utility. Under such circumstances, this well gotten up drama of importation may be rehearsed in every epidemic, adapted in all its parts to every place and every disease, they wish to make contagious. First will be presented, as at Gibraltar, the actual importers— their course traced—the disease identified—its reception denounced, and quarantine established; and this will go down until sober minded disinterested men become engaged in the enquiry, when it will turn out in all probability, that the importers, as at Sunderland, never had the disease— that it was in the place long before their arrival—that in its supposed course, it either had no existence, or had long ceased—in fact that the importation was a fable, the product either of design or an alarmed imagination. On this point I shall not here farther dwell, but proceed to the still keenly disputed question of its contagious, or non-contagious nature.

Amongst all those who have advocated the affirmative side of the question, an anonymous writer in the LANCET, of Nov. 19th. seems to me the ablest special pleader of his party, and the best informed on the subject, which he has grappled with a degree of acumen and power that must at once have secured him the victory, in any cause that had truth for its basis, or that could have stood by itself; but strong and scornful as he is, he has himself furnished the weapons for his own defeat, and has only to be correctly quoted in his own words, for answer to the most imposing and powerful of his arguments. I take it for granted, that no one will give credit to instantaneous infection, at first sight, but allow that an interval must elapse between the reception of the virus, and explosion of the disease. Kennedy and the best of the contagionist authors, have fixed the intervening time from two days to a longer uncertain period; yet that writer (in the LANCET) proceeds to tell us, in proof of the virulence of the contagion, that when twenty healthy reapers went into the harvest field at Swedia, near Tripoli, and one of them at mid-day was struck down with the disease, he then instantly, as if, instead of being prostrate on the ground, he had run a muck for the propagation of Cholera Morbus, infected all the rest, so that the whole were down within three hours, and all were dead before the following morning.[29]—All this too in the open air. Another writer of note relates that when a healthy ship on the outward voyage arrived in Madras Roads, her people were seized with Cholera Morbus that very morning; but they go further than this, and command us to believe in its contagious powers, without sight at all, quoting the report from our Commissioners in Russia, where it is officially announced "that neither the presence, nor contact of the patient is necessary to communicate the disease." Surely in candour we may be allowed to say that when they limit their views to contagion alone, they have attributed powers to it, which it never did, and never can possess. That some other principle, besides their favourite one, must have been in operation, as well in the field of Swedia, when it struck down the reapers, as when it blighted our armies in the East, for these sudden bursts and explosions of pestilence are incompatible with the laws and progress of natural contagion,—that if, under a tropical temperature, which dissipates all infection, there be contagion in the disease, their must also be other powers of diffusion hitherto inscrutable, incomprehensible, and uncontroulable,—that their doctrine of contagion exclusively, is superficial narrow, and intolerant, and their arguments in support of it, no more than a delusion of prejudice, a piece of consummate special pleading to make the worse appear the better reason.[30]

[29] The precise words are "20 peasants of Swedia, robust, vigorous, and in the flower of life, were labouring at the harvest work, when on the 9th. of July, at noon, one was suddenly attacked, and the others in a short time showed symptoms of the disorder. In three hours, the entire band was exhausted; before sunset many had ceased to live, and by the morrow there was no survivor."

[30] The remainder of the paper, as presented to the Society, treated of Typhus fever, and other matter, that had no reference to the disease in question.

Before concluding these observations, I would wish to make a few remarks upon some points of the enquiry which have been either too cursorily passed over, or not noticed at all; and first of its supposed attraction for, and adherence to the lines and courses of rivers whether navigable or otherwise. I do not think this quality of the disease has been assumed on grounds sufficient to justify anything like an exclusive preference. Along these lines, no doubt, it has very frequently been found, because a malarious, a terrestrial, a contagious, or indeed any other disease, would for many reasons, best prevail on the lowest levels of the country, or the deepest lines on its surface, like the vallies of rivers, provided the food on which it fed—population—there abounded. It would be difficult almost anywhere to point out a populous city unconnected with the sea, rivers, or canals, the water population of which, from their habits of life and occupations, everywhere crowded, dirty, careless, and exposed, must always afford ready materials for any epidemic to work upon, and this may have given currency to the prevailing opinion; but I rather believe, when enquiry comes to be made, it will be found that the worst ravages of Cholera Morbus have been experienced in the great level open plains of Upper Germany, and the boundless jungly districts of India, remote from, or at least unconnected with water communication, denoting thereby atmospheric influence and agency, rather than any other.

Another consideration of some importance is the burial of the dead, which according to published reports, has in some places been enforced in so hurried a manner as deeply to wound the feelings of surviving relatives, and in others to give rise to the horrid suspicion of premature interment. Can this have been necessary in any disease, even allowing it to be contagious, or was it wise and dignified in the medical profession to make this concession to popular prejudice, at all times when excited, so unmanageable and troublesome. Although we cannot analyse the matter of contagion, we surely know enough of it to feel assured, that it must be a production and exhalation from the living body, arising out of certain processes going on there, in other words out of the disease itself, which disease must cease along with the life of the patient, and the exhalation be furnished no longer—that during life it was sublimed, so as to leave the body and become diffused around through the agency of the animal heat, created by the functions of respiration and circulation of the blood, which being foreclosed and the supplies cut off, all that remained of it floating before death in the atmosphere, must be condensed upon the cold corpse and lie harmless.[31] It must also be evident that when putrefaction begins, no production of what belonged to the living body can remain unchanged, but must undergo the transformation in form, substance and quality, ordained for all things; for putrefaction, although it may possibly produce a disease after its own character, is not pestilence, nor even compatible with it in the case of specific diseases.

[31] Even when a living product, we are authorised to believe, from observations made upon the plague, that it cannot be propelled to a greater distance than a few feet from the body of the patient—that it is heavier than common air, settling down in a remarkable manner upon the sick bed, and saturating the lower strata of the atmosphere in the sick apartment.

The puerile stories, therefore, of infection being taken from following a coffined corpse to the grave, without reference to the state of grief, fear, and fatigue, not improbably, of drunkenness, in the mourners, must be unworthy of attention. I am no friend to the absurdly long interval which in this country is allowed to elapse,[32] even in the hottest weather, between death and burial; but still more do I deprecate the indecent haste which would give sanction to panic, and incur the risk or even the suspicion of interment
before dissolution. In regard to separate burying grounds, should the disease come to spread, I am sure no one will expect, after what has just been said, that I should attempt to argue the question seriously, nor enter a protest against the further gratuitous wrong of withholding the rites of sepulture in consecrated ground from the victims of an epidemic or even a contagious disease.—Nothing could warrant such a measure but want of room in the ordinary churchyards, where police should never be allowed to interfere with the rights and feelings or property, of the living, unless to ensure the privacy of funerals; nothing being so appalling to an alarmed people as the spectacle of death in their streets, or so trying to the health of the mourners, as tedious funeral ceremonies amidst a crowd of people.

[32] After sending these letters to the press, I saw in the public prints that the Bishop of the Diocese had forbidden the funerals of the dead from Cholera to be received in the churches of London. Instead of thus forbidding a part, better have the whole of the service performed there (where crowds do not come) under cover from the weather, than in the open churchyard, where the mourners uncovered, are exposed in every way to damp and cold, and the jostling of the mob; better still have all the service deemed necessary, performed at the residence of the deceased.

Were I called upon to criticise what I have now written, and to review all that I have seen, read, and heard on the subject, I would conscientiously declare that the importation of Cholera Morbus into England or anywhere else, had been clearly negatived, and its non-contagious character almost as clearly established, always however with the proviso and exception of the possibility of its being made a temporary contingent contagion, amidst filth and poverty, and impurity of atmosphere, from overcrowding and accumulation of sick, but neither transmissible nor transportable out of its own locality, through human intercourse. As the disease, like all the other great plagues, which at various periods have desolated the earth, evidently came from the east, it would be most desirable in pursuing our investigation, to have a clear knowledge of the mode of its introduction into Russia on the eastern boundary of Europe. Unfortunately we can place no dependence upon the reports that have been published to prove importation there, which are lame and contradictory, although coming from the avowed partizans of contagion; but even had they been better gotten up, we could not, unless they had been confirmed by the experience of other nations, have received them with implicit reliance.

The Russian Employé of the provinces, *mendacior Parthis*, not from greater innate moral depravity than others, but from the corruptions of a despotic government which compel him to live under the rod of a master, amidst a superstitious barbarous population, whose dangerous prejudices he dare not offend, can only give utterance to what his tyrants command. Even at the more civilized capital of Petersburgh, the mob rose in arms to murder the foreign physicians when they did not act according to their liking. Could the truth then be heard on such a field, or what native officer would venture to impugn the authority of his rulers, proclaiming contagion? If he did, he must cease to live in the official sense of the word. Throughout Europe, from east to west, the disease has followed its own route according to its own incomprehensible laws, despite of every obstacle and precaution. We have the authority of our own Central Board for believing that the disease cannot be conveyed by merchandize of any kind, and that of our mission to Russia for greatly doubting whether it can adhere to personal clothing or bedding; and will it be pretended that human beings, labouring under such a distemper in any form, could have been the vehicles of spreading it in a straight line for thousands of miles throughout civilized nations, armed and prepared to defend themselves against its inroads,— they tried, but in vain. We, too, may strive to discover the demon of the pestilence amidst the clouds of the climate, or the winds of Heaven. He remains hidden to our view; and until better revealed, it only remains for us to exercise towards our fellow men those duties which humanity prompts, civilization teaches, and religion enjoins.

POSTSCRIPT.

My friend, Doctor Stanford, of the Medical Staff, now settled here, has given me the following valuable information, which my own observation confirms, regarding the agency of panic, in promoting the diffusion of epidemic disease. He happened to be serving with part of the British army, at Cadiz, when an eruption of yellow fever took place there, in the autumn of 1813, and as usually happens amongst medical men, the first time they have seen that fever, some of them were staunch contagionists, and impressed that belief upon the corps to which they belonged. In all these the disease was most fatal to great numbers. The men being half dead with fear, before they were taken ill, speedily became its victims, to the great terror and danger of their surviving comrades; but in the other regiments, where no alarm had been sounded, the soldiers took the chances of the epidemic with the same steady courage they would have faced the bullets of the enemy, in the lottery of battle; escaping an attack for the most part altogether, or if seized, recovering from it in a large proportion. From this picture let us take a lesson, in case the impending epidemic should ever come to spread in the populous towns of England, and the cry of contagion be proclaimed in their streets. The very word will spread terror and dismay throughout the people, causing multitudes to be infected, who would otherwise, in all probability, have escaped an attack, and afterwards consign them to death in despair, when they find themselves the marked and fated victims of a new plague. Whatever they see around them, must confirm and aggravate their despair, for desertion and excommunication in all dangerous diseases, too certainly seal the fate of the patient. It will be vain to tell them that hireling attendance has been provided,—the life of the Choleraic depends upon the instant aid—the able bodied willing aid of affectionate friends, who will devote themselves to the task, and persevere indefatigably to the last. If these be driven from his bed, his last stay is gone, for without their active co-operation the best prescription of the physician is only so much waste paper. What, let me ask, must have been the fate of the patient, and what the consequent panic, if the case of Cholera that occurred in London, a month ago at the Barracks of the Foot Guards, had been proclaimed, and treated as a contagion? The poor fellow was promptly surrounded by his fearless comrades, who with their kind hands recalled and preserved the vital heat on the surface, by persevering in the affectionate duty of rubbing him for many hours; but had the Medical Staff of the regiment been true contagionists, they must, as in duty bound, have commanded, and compelled every one of them to fly the infection. It depended upon them, to have spread around a far wilder and more dangerous contagion than that of Cholera Morbus, or any other disease,— the contagion of fear—and from what occurred at Cadiz, as above related, it is to be hoped our medical men will now see how much they will have it in their power, when Cholera comes, to pronounce, or to withhold sentence of desolation upon a community. The word Contagion will be the word of doom, for then the healthy will fly their homes, and the sick be deserted; but a countenance and bearing, devoid of that groundless fear, will at once command the aid, and inspire the hopes that are powerful to save in the most desperate diseases.

It is stated, in a Scotch newspaper, that two poor travellers, passing from Kirkintulloch to Falkirk, ran the risque of being stoned to death by the populace of the latter place, and were saved from the immolation only by escaping into a house; and in an Irish one, that some shipwrecked sailors incurred a similar danger. Such barbarities must, in the nature of things, be practised every where under a reign of terror, however humane or christianized the people may be—even the fatalism of the Turk would not be proof against it. In Spain they have been enacted in all their horrors (thanks to the quarantine laws) upon the unfortunate victims of yellow fever;[33] and we shall soon see them repeated amongst ourselves, unless the plain truth be promulgated by authority to the people. Let them be told if such be the pleasure of our rulers, (for it is not worth while disputing the point), that Cholera Morbus is a contagion, but of so safe a nature in regard to communicability, that not one in a hundred, or even a thousand, take the disease,—that in this country, besides being a transient passing disease, which according to certain laws and peculiarities of its own, will assuredly take its departure in no long time; it is limited almost always to particular spots and localities—that it is in their own power, while it remains, to correct the infectious atmosphere of these spots, by attention to health police—that they may fearlessly approach their sick friends with impunity, for that the danger resides in the above atmosphere, and not in the person of the patient; and that in all situations they may defy it, for as long as they observe sobriety of life and regularity of habits. Thus will public confidence be restored, and thus be verified the homely adage of, "honesty, in all human affairs, being ever the best policy"; for the concealment, or perversion of the truth, however much it may be made to serve the purposes of the passing day, can never ultimately promote the ends of good government and true humanity, but must lead, sooner or later, to the exposure of the delusion, or what would be far worse, to the perpetuation of error and prejudice, and grossest abuse of the people, in regard to those interests committed to our charge.

[33] Vide O'Halloran, upon the Yellow Fever in Spain.

Doctor Henry, of Manchester, has, in a late paper, published some most interesting experiments, upon the disinfecting power of heat. He found that the vaccine virus was deprived of its infecting quality, at 140° of Farenheit, and that the contagions of Scarlatina, and Typhus fever, from fomites, were certainly dissipated and destroyed, at the dry heat of boiling water. In regard to these last, he might surely have ventured to fix the standard of safety at a greatly lower temperature; for if the grosser vaccine matter could be rendered inert at 140°, there can be little doubt of the subtile gaseous emanations, which constitute the aerial contagions, being dissipated by the same agent, at an inferior degree. In the absence of direct experiment, we may venture to infer, that 120° would suffice, to nullify these last. Such, at least, has been the belief of those, who have been employed to purify ships, barracks, and hospitals, from contagion, and I should think it must have been founded on experience.[34]

[34] As far back as the years 1796-7-8, this fact was familiar to us in the St. Domingo war, only we were satisfied with a minimum heat of 120°, from a belief that a temperature of that height, as it coagulated the ova of insects (the cock roach for instance), and was otherwise incompatible with insect life, would avail to dissipate contagion.

He does not treat of the disinfecting property of light, although such an agent was well worthy of his notice; for the power, which in closely stopped bottles can deprive Cayenne Pepper of its sting—render our Prussic Acid as harmless as cream, and convert the strongest medicinal powders into so much powder of *post*, can also avail to destroy the matter and principle of Contagion. In fact, no other is used for purifying goods, at our Lazzarettoes, where suspected articles of merchandise, after some nugatory fumigations, are simply exposed to light and air with such certain effect, that there is not, I believe, in this country, any record of infection being propagated from them afterwards. The experiments of Doctor Henry are as simple and beautiful in themselves, as they promise to be useful and important, for now even the horrible contagion of hospital gangrene would appear to be under the controul of the pure agent he has been describing; and the principle now established of light and heat, the grand vivifying powers of the creation, being the sure and true preservers of the creature, man, from the poisons generated even by himself, and otherwise around him, calls for our admiration and gratitude, as shewing that these agents and emanations of Almighty power can be made, in the hands of the practical philosopher, to serve the purposes of domestic science, and in as far as we can see, to fulfil, at least in that respect, the best intentions of the Creator.

PART I

Foot 1: Removed stray comma (As medical men in this Country employ)

Page 6: Changed possesss to possess (still do not possess)

Page 13: Removed superfluous quote marks (Petersburg;—this gentleman)

Page 19: Removed duplicate word 'of' (has become a magazine of)

Page 19: Changed . to , (the cause of cholera,)

Page 21: Changed , to . (&c., in the office)

Page 22: Changed Mauritus to Mauritius (at the Mauritius before)

Page 22: Added . to Dr (Dr. Hawkins admits)

Page 24: Changed . to , (Martin M'Neal[6],)

Page 24: Changed knowlege to knowledge (any knowledge himself)

Page 26: Changed circustances to circumstances (two circumstances)

Page 28: Removed duplicate word 'a' (at least for a time)

Page 32: Changed intercouse to intercourse (or great intercourse)

Page 33: Added . to Dr (and Dr. Hawkins)

Foot 11: Changed importan to important (in the important)

Page 39: Moved misplaced comma (at Barcelonetta, the)

Page 45: Changed teminated to terminated (terminated favourably)

Page 46: Removed stray hyphen (he persists in giving)

Page 50: Moved misplaced period (this calamity (the cholera).)

Page 51: Changed çaon to 'ça on' (toute ça on trouve)

Page 53: Deleted superfluous end-quotes (took place.)

Page 53: Changed confied to confined (been confined to her bed)

Page 53: Changed macron to aigu accent (employés attached)

Page 53: Changed authorties to authorities (authorities wished)

Page 54: Changed dimished to diminished (diminished all at once)

Page 54: Changed á to à (tout à coup)

Page 54: Changed entassès to entassés (crowded [entassés])

Page 54: Changed Franec to France (state like France)

Page 56: Added missing end-quotes (to the Burraumposter.")

Page 57: Changed em-dash to hyphen (Leicester-square)

PART II

Page 11: Changed typhoi'd to typhoid (the typhoid principle)

Page 15: Changed affluuent to affluent (houses of the affluent)

Page 17: Changed 'in' to 'In' (in my last letter)

Page 21: Changed absorded to absorbed (absorbed into the soil)

Page 22: Changed 'in' to 'it' (would certainly have kept it)

Page 24: Changed procees to process (drying process)

Page 26: Changed saered to sacred (the most sacred duty)

Page 30: Added missing ending punctuation (following morning.)

Page 31: Removed duplicate word always (always afford)

CPSIA information can be obtained
at www.ICGtesting.com
Printed in the USA
LVHW030140271222
735871LV00001B/259

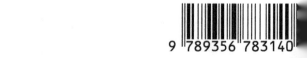

9 789356 783140